Breast Cancer:

What You Should Know (But May Not Be Told) About Prevention, Diagnosis, and Treatment

◆

Steve Austin, N.D.
Cathy Hitchcock, M.S.W.

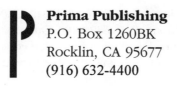

Prima Publishing
P.O. Box 1260BK
Rocklin, CA 95677
(916) 632-4400

Please note: Our purpose is to facilitate and in no way replace doctor-patient interactions. This book serves to educate—not to diagnose or treat breast cancer. All attempts have been made to ensure that the contents are accurate at the time of publication.

Library of Congress Cataloging-in-Publication Data

Austin, Steve,
   Breast cancer : what you should know (but may not be told) about
prevention, diagnosis, and treatment / Steve Austin, Cathy Hitchcock.
      p.   cm.
   Includes bibliographical references and index.
   ISBN 1-55958-362-2 (pbk.)
   1. Breast—Cancer—Popular works.   I. Hitchcock, Cathy,
II. Title.
   RC280.B8A93   1994
   616.99'449—dc20   93-49716
                                                                    CIP

97   98   **AA**   10   9   8

Printed in the United States of America

How to Order:
Single copies may be ordered from Prima Publishing, P.O. Box 1260BK, Rocklin, CA 95667; telephone (916) 632-4400. Quantity discounts are also available. On your letterhead, include information concerning the intended use of the books and the number of books you wish to purchase.

Austin and Hitchcock skillfully blend intense personal experience and a searching, comprehensively documented analysis and evaluation of all types of breast cancer therapy, "conventional" and "alternative." A must-read for anyone interested in the prevention and treatment of breast cancer, and the story of one woman's path to wholeness and wellness.

—Johnathan V. Wright, M.D.
author of *Dr. Wright's Guide to Healing with Nutrition*

◆

This is the best breast book ever! Remarkably written and researched, it includes both the patient's and doctor's points of view and should be required reading for everyone.

—Sandra McClanahan, M.D.
Director of Stress Management Training at
Dean Ornish's Preventive Medicine Institute
author of the forthcoming *Whole Surgery Handbook* (1995)

◆

Comprehensive, accurate, and readable. . . . Austin and Hitch-cock have done a great service with this book, and I will recommend it to patients and families faced with this terrible disease.

—Andrew Weil, M.D.
author of *Spontaneous Healing*

◆

A must for any breast cancer patient. This is the only book that gives women the opportunity to evaluate both conventional and alternative approaches in making their own informed decisions.

—Michael Murray, N.D.
author of *Encyclopedia of Natural Medicine*

◆

This upbeat book offers practical suggestions for women coping with various stages of breast cancer. The book is also valuable for all who wish to take control of their lives for good health . . . .

—Beatrice Trum Hunter
food editor, *Consumers' Research* Magazine

To Dr. John Bastyr,
the father of modern naturopathic medicine

C O N T E N T S

PART 4 *Living with Breast Cancer*   267

Foreword

According to current statistics, as many as one of every eight American women will develop breast cancer. That percentage has been steadily increasing, despite the best that modern medicine has to offer.

Few if any diseases invoke more fear and distrust than does cancer. Conventional treatment—primarily chemotherapy, radiation, and surgery—leaves a lot to be desired in terms of both effectiveness and safety. Alternative medicine, which offers diets, nutritional supplements, herbs, and other modalities, is obviously less toxic than conventional therapy. However, if these treatments do not work, then choosing them over conventional approaches could be dangerous.

In this book, Dr. Steve Austin has done a beautiful job of clarifying much of the confusion and controversy related to preventing and treating breast cancer. Although one might expect a naturopathic physician to be biased against conventional treatments and toward natural remedies, Dr. Austin has clearly left any potential bias at home. I have known Dr. Austin for more than ten years and have always been impressed by his ability to sift through mountains of conflicting data in his search for the truth. When Steve Austin tells me something about medicine, I rarely feel the need to look it up myself. More important, he has never been afraid to report his findings, no matter whose belief systems they might threaten.

Conventional medicine has been criticized for being too dangerous, too expensive, and too often ineffective. These criticisms are sometimes well deserved. Nevertheless, surgery, chemotherapy, and radiation have saved the lives of thousands of breast cancer patients. Natural medicine and other alternatives are appealing, and there are good reasons for recommending dietary changes, nutritional supplements, and other non-toxic modalities. However, in certain situations, these treatments should be used in addition to, rather than instead of, conventional therapy.

Austin combines an exhaustive review of the medical literature with a good deal of common sense to provide you with useful guidelines. When is lumpectomy preferable to mastectomy? When is it necessary to remove the axillary lymph nodes? Should you have radiation therapy? Should you take vitamin and mineral supplements and change your diet? Dr. Austin does not presume to tell you what is best for you, because these decisions are yours to make and to live with. However, he provides you with the information you need to break through the superstition (in both conventional and alternative medicine) and make informed choices.

Cathy Hitchcock is a survivor of breast cancer who chose her own path to recovery. Her story, intertwined with the scientific research reviewed by her husband, provides an important perspective. Hitchcock gives a personal account of how she made the decision to go against her doctor's advice by having a lumpectomy *without* lymph node dissection and radiation. She also describes the ways in which she sought to heal her life, through diet, visualization, and various naturopathic remedies. Hitchcock is not a rebel, but she is unwilling to submit to doctors' orders unless they are consistent with scientific research and with her personal philosophy.

Breast Cancer: What You Should Know (But May Not Be Told) About Prevention, Diagnosis, and Treatment is a landmark book and important reading for anyone who has or who is interested in preventing this dread disease.

Alan R. Gaby, M.D.
President, American Holistic Medical Association

Acknowledgments

Writing this book has been a team effort.

Thank you is too small a phrase for the many hours our dear friends Blaze Newman and Barbara Branscomb spent improving our manuscript from its inception to completion.

Our thanks to National College of Naturopathic Medicine for its support and especially to President Timothy Duszynski, Ph.D., and Jared Zeff, N.D., former Academic Dean. Steve also thanks his breast cancer patients at the Portland Naturopathic Clinic for constantly reminding him that this is not an academic project—it involves real people.

We are grateful to our literary agent, Natasha Kern, for believing in our book, guiding us through the intricacies of writing a book proposal, sending us relevant articles and books to read, and most of all, getting us a contract with Prima Publishing. We also are indebted to her for suggesting Louise Nelson as a publicist whose enthusiastic support is a writer's dream.

Prima Publishing has been the perfect match for our book. We thank Jennifer Basye, Karen Blanco, and Jenn Nelson for their spirited support. Most of all, we thank our editor, Andi Reese Brady, whose help and expertise have been available to us through thick and thin.

We hold in high regard the fine editing help of Jane Gilligan at Bookman Productions and the eagle eye of Joan Pendleton.

We are also thankful for the editing of our initial chapters by friends Gretchen Newmark, R.D., Joanne Fuller, M.S.W., Karen Boyle, R.N., M.A., Jan McMurphey, M.A., and Kris Falco, Psy.D.

We thank Beatrice Trum Hunter for her inspiration over the years and for her ninth inning help.

Nick Soloway, L.M.T., D.C., L.Ac., spent countless hours at the medical libraries keeping Steve supplied with the latest breast cancer research. Lyn Scott's quality secretarial help and computer knowledge were critical at early stages of the project. We appreciate your efforts.

We offer thanks to Joseph Pizzorno, N.D., Jim Sensenig, N.D., Jan Bernard, R.N., Bob Timberlake and the Institute for Naturopathic Medicine, and dear friend Skye Lininger, D.C., who have all given critical support at pivotal moments.

Steve thanks Jonathan V. Wright, M.D., and Alan R. Gaby, M.D.—mentors, teachers, and friends who have pioneered the serious study of clinical nutrition without conventional allopathic biases.

Cathy thanks Bob Martin, D.S.W., for his psychological genius and Tom Stokes, Ph.D., for his mastery of guided imagery. She may be alive and well today to write this book because of their help.

Last, but not least, we thank and cherish our many friends and family not named here who have enthusiastically supported our writing despite seeing much less of us these past three years.

Introduction

You've found the lump. You're frightened. What do you do?

This book asks women to take back the power to make their own decisions—decisions that go beyond the choices they are typically given by their oncologists, surgeons, or popular books. These decisions may literally save the lives of some of the 186,000 American women who will be diagnosed with breast cancer this year.

We're writing for women who choose to actively participate in their diagnosis and treatment—not for those who want someone to tell them what to do.

Most books for women with breast cancer are written by doctors who advocate or patients who are using conventional treatments exclusively. But a wealth of information in the medical library is now being ignored by conventional medicine. Much of it is also neglected by both alternative medicine and popular books on breast cancer. We provide this information to allow you to make informed decisions and question your doctor's advice in an intelligent way. You have every right to question conventional medicine. In the United States, the death rate from breast cancer is no better now than it was a half century ago.

Such a skeptical attitude in itself might actually enhance a woman's chance of survival. One research group found that long-term survivors of breast cancer had "a more negative attitude" toward their conventional treatment and "significantly poorer attitudes" toward their physicians;[1] that is, they became active, questioning participants in their diagnosis and treatment.

We're also writing for the millions of women who want to prevent breast cancer. The *Journal of the National Cancer Institute* now says the overall lifetime risk for developing breast cancer is one in eight for American women.[2] A high level of education, eating a typical American diet, being childless, a family history of breast cancer, or being Jewish all put you at greater risk. So does an early first menstrual period or menopause after age 50. For the millions at risk, this book may offer protection from ever having to face the shock of a breast cancer diagnosis.

Step-by-step, we walk the reader through each part of diagnosis, treatment (both conventional and alternative), and prevention (including prevention of a recurrence) with the help of a diagnostic flow chart, questions to ask the doctor, checklists, summaries, and overviews.

Interwoven with all this information, Cathy shares her personal story as a breast cancer patient. She describes her ordeal upon discovering the lump and the transitions she has gone through to live with the diagnosis in a life-affirming way. Unlike many other breast cancer patients, Cathy didn't simply accept the choices offered by medical doctors. Instead, she studied the research we describe in this book and made her own decisions about conventional and alternative treatments.

Steve is an N.D.—naturopathic doctor. Naturopathic physicians employ most of the same diagnostic tools used by medical doctors but treat with nutrition, supplements, herbs, manipulation, hydrotherapy, and other natural therapies. Steve covers both conventional and alternative treatment approaches, but his viewpoint differs from that of conventional medicine: Naturopathic doctors facilitate the body's innate ability to heal, rather than focus on the removal of symptoms. Sometimes natural approaches should not be used to the exclusion of conventional medical treatments. Therefore, naturopathic physicians frequently refer patients to medical doctors. Naturopaths are licensed in Oregon, Washington, Montana, Hawaii, Alaska, Arizona, Connecticut, and most Canadian provinces. Naturopathy is also practiced in many states where licensing doesn't exist.

Medical doctors often interpret the research on surgery, radiation, chemotherapy, and tamoxifen through the lens of conventional medical philosophy. A chemotherapy study that shows a tiny advantage may be heralded as a breakthrough, even though most patients don't benefit and all suffer the consequences of the treatment.

Even more harmful to the patient is the fact that nonscientific factors can play a role in how medical knowledge is applied. Many more mastectomies and fewer lumpectomies are performed in the South than in other areas of the country.[3] Obviously, this has nothing to do with science. Information in *Breast Cancer: What You Should Know (But May Not Be Told) About Prevention, Diagnosis, and Treatment* gives a woman in Alabama the same treatment choices as a woman in Connecticut.

Conventional medical philosophy often takes precedence over science. Even well-intentioned medical doctors' interpretations of the research can leave you with a view contradictory to the one you would develop if you read the research. We make you aware of and help you understand the research, enabling you to participate in decisions that may affect your survival.

Some subjects, like nutritional supplements, are simply taboo for many oncologists. Not here. Our book evaluates alternative treatments. Other books on alternative therapies have often dangled hope irresponsibly before desperate patients. Treatments that a few surviving patients have undergone are made to sound like common cures, although no scientific support is provided. Steve led a research project in Mexico following patients who attended alternative clinics. Most of these treatments didn't work. Our section on alternative therapies provides information on which are worthy of consideration.

Psychological intervention can increase the chances for breast cancer survival, yet many medical doctors downplay research supporting this fact. We give it the space it deserves and suggest how you can use this information to live longer.

You needn't read the whole book at once. And don't feel you need to read it in the sequence presented. Jump to the chapter that covers a decision immediately in front of you. If you have two days to decide about chemotherapy, read the sections about chemo first. If you have breast cancer, we understand what you are going through—we have been going through it ourselves.

Today, about 80 percent of breast cancer patients are diagnosed at an early stage. "Early stage" (stages I and II, in medical jargon) means relatively limited disease and, therefore, an excellent chance of surviving many years and dying of something unrelated. This book is geared for early-stage breast cancer patients and for women trying to prevent the disease. Conventional treatment of and prognosis for later stages will not be discussed. However, late-stage patients may find our chapter on alternative treatments especially useful.

Breast Cancer: What You Should Know (But May Not Be Told) About Prevention, Diagnosis, and Treatment is not an attempt to show you how to treat cancer, let alone diagnose yourself. Treatment decisions must be tailored to the individual patient. We encourage you to discuss the information in this book with your doctor(s) before making any decisions. If your current doctor doesn't wish to discuss anything but "party-line" medicine, consider getting a second opinion. It's your body, it's your life, and it's your nickel.

References

1. Derogatis, L. R., M. D. Abeloff, and N. Melisaratos. Psychological coping mechanisms and survival time in metastatic breast cancer. *JAMA* 1979;242:1504–8.

2. Feuer, E. J. et al. The lifetime risk of developing breast cancer. *J Natl Cancer Inst* 1993;85:892–6.

3. Nattinger, A. B., et al. Geographic variation in the use of breast-conserving treatment for breast cancer. *N Engl J Med* 1992;326:1102–7.

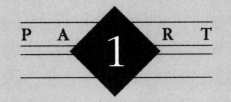

Diagnostic Choices

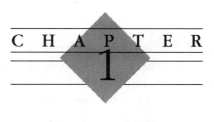

Shock

CATHY

In 1972 I was on the trip of a lifetime. I had been traveling in Europe for eight months with my first husband, Bill, on a journey to heal the psychic wounds after his return from Vietnam. That spring he was driving the car on a mountain road in Greece as we headed for Delphi; I remember we had been joking about going to see the oracle. We never made it. As we rounded a bend, we saw a concrete guardrail ahead that looked like the only protection a skidding car would have to keep it from falling off the mountain. Unfortunately, we were in a skidding car; it was raining after weeks of sunshine, and the road was slick. Even worse, part of the guardrail was missing — the part we were sliding toward at 30 miles per hour. It had already been knocked out by another car in exactly the same predicament. We had no idea what lay beyond it — a drop of 10 feet or 1,000. The time it took from the moment I realized we were going through the concrete guard to God-only-knew-where and when it actually happened was probably a matter of 5 or 10 seconds. It seemed like a very long time. I was paralyzed with fear. I knew I was going to die. I wanted to tell Bill that I loved him, but I couldn't speak. He was able to say something, slowly, with the most agony I have ever heard in anybody's voice: "Oh, my God!"

We broke through the guardrail. The car dropped about 20 feet and flipped over. I remember thinking, "Please, God, let it stop now, and we'll live." And then it flipped again. And then again. We were now about 300 feet down the mountain. All four

3

doors had flown off, and the glass had popped out. Everything in the car except Bill and me was now spread over the mountainside. I had been wearing my seat belt. The direction of the roll threw Bill against me, and my belt held us both in the car. It was a junky little Renault 10 that had been a lemon from the moment we picked it up; but it had roll bars, and they worked when we really needed them.

I was paralyzed from the waist down. Bill, covered with bruises, crawled up the mountain and scaled a 20-foot cliff at the top to wave down the first car that came by. The car was filled with a Greek family, also on their way to Delphi. They emptied out their car, leaving most of the family standing in the rain. They made a makeshift stretcher and brought me up the hill. They turned the car around and took Bill and me to a hospital 20 miles away. The driver didn't leave until he knew we were going to be okay.

I will always love the Greeks.

A few hours later, the shock wore off; I was no longer paralyzed. I suffered cuts, abrasions, and some whiplash, but no broken bones. I was going to be fine. The trauma was over and I could begin to heal.

Seventeen years later, in February 1989, during a self-exam, I discovered a lump in my breast. I mentioned it to a good friend while on a weekend trip to Seattle. She remembers my saying, "I'm not going to think about something so unpleasant when we're here to have fun." I simply forgot about it. A month later, I noticed the lump as if for the first time and mentioned it casually to my husband, Steve. The lump worried him, and he pushed me to set up an appointment with my naturopathic doctor and arrange for a mammogram. I probably would have forgotten about it again if he hadn't been so concerned.

I went to my naturopathic doctor and waited for her to tell me it was just another fibrocystic lump. She agreed it might be and said we could follow it. Only when I mentioned that Steve thought I should get a mammogram did she say it could be arranged.

I went to an outpatient clinic to have a mammogram — my first. It can be compared to having a pelvic exam: unpleasant and a bit unnerving. The technician told me that the mammogram was inconclusive and that the radiologist would come to my dressing room to discuss it. The radiologist told me basically the same thing: that we could "follow it" — a phrase I've come to dislike. Then, just as he was about to leave, he mentioned that we could do an ultrasound if I really wanted to. I asked him what this procedure would achieve; he explained that sometimes tumors show up on ultrasound when they can't be seen on the mammogram. We wouldn't know whether it was benign or malignant, but we would know whether it was a solid tumor or a cyst. I asked, "Why wait?" He said the expense was the main reason. When I asked him about the cost, he said that it would be under $100. So I pushed a bit and was able to have the ultrasound done that day.

The ultrasound tech called in the radiologist to have a look. He took a cursory glance and said that it all looked cystic; everything was going to be okay. As he started to leave the room, the technician pointed to a *solid* spot on the screen.

Then the radiologist gave me a little talk about how most of these lumps are benign, probably nothing to worry about. He told me that I should just put it out of my mind until I went in for the biopsy. I heard all of this distantly as if through thick cotton batting. I was in shock.

It was a lot like the other time, on that road in Greece. This time I was able to talk. But it wasn't really me talking to the doctor. I was far away. I had that same sinking feeling I had had as I went toward the hole in the guardrail — I knew I was going to die.

I had gone to both my naturopathic doctor and the mammogram clinic to be reassured, to rule out the unmentionable and be told everything was fine. The doctors were all too eager to accommodate me. If I hadn't pushed all the way, it would have been left at that. It seemed the doctors hadn't wanted to find out that I had cancer either — they were all for "following it."

I hadn't had the foresight to have Steve go with me. After all, we had had no experience with this situation. I remember driving home and feeling as if I were in a surrealistic movie. How could other people just drive along as if they had their whole lives in front of them, when mine might be behind me? I felt disconnected from my body. As I walked in the front door of our house, I remembered that our bedroom was being wallpapered. The sweet man who was doing this job was pleased because it was turning out beautifully. When he came out of the bedroom with a big smile on his face and saw me, his smile disappeared. I had thought I was hiding my feelings. (I don't know why I always think I can do this, but somehow, in the moment, it seems possible.) He asked me what had happened, and I told him. He hugged me, and I cried. I was glad he was there, but I couldn't handle the feelings. The shock took over again. I left the house, drove to an unfamiliar restaurant, and ordered a margarita with lunch. I think I ordered a second drink.

I wanted to numb out.

In Greece, a few hours after the accident, the shock started to wear off and the paralysis left. In Portland, a few hours after the ultrasound, the shock was just revving up and there seemed to be no end in sight.

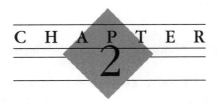

My Diagnosis

CATHY

My mind is racing. My emotions are in turmoil. One moment I'm feeling like a zombie; the next I'm in a panic. Underneath it all is a sinking feeling telling me I'm going to die. Before my time. Soon.

In this irrational state I'm required to make perhaps the most important decisions of my life. I need to think clearly. I have to choose a doctor and decide whether to do a needle biopsy, excision biopsy, or lumpectomy (see pages 15–17). I am an emotional basket case; after all, I know in my gut it is cancer and that I'm going to die, so what's the point? Steve takes over. I realize how lucky I am to have someone close who is familiar with the latest research on breast cancer. Unfortunately, few people have this luxury.

My family doctor, a naturopath, recommends a couple of surgeons. Friends recommend a few more. Steve spends a day on the phone screening surgeons. The doctor he is most pleased with is not a "Blue Cross Preferred Provider." Because my policy offers good coverage only for "preferred providers," I would get a mere 60 percent reimbursement with this doctor. So, we rule her out because we have no idea what our medical bills may come to, except some fantasy that screams "bankruptcy!" We opt for a "preferred provider."

Although I haven't even seen a doctor yet, we've come up against some of the financial problems of our medical-insurance system, and we have made our first crucial decision based on

7

financial fears rather than on medical preference. Nothing like a
little added stress.

The doctor we choose gets us in right away, which is both
relieving and scary. I'll get more information, but will it be what I
want to hear?

We go to the appointment. The doctor palpates my breast,
reassuring me that he has felt hundreds of lumps and that this
doesn't feel like cancer. He can usually "tell by the feel," but we
should do a biopsy* "just in case." I'm feeling immensely relieved.
Steve is with me while the doctor does the biopsy in his office. I
feel very brave. Usually I'm squeamish about such things, but I
come through this ordeal like a pro. The doctor cuts out the
tumor, says he is sure it's benign by its appearance, and discards
the half that's usually tested for estrogen receptor status (see page
24) — he is that sure. He says he'll give us a call on Thursday
with the results, but not to worry; he is practically positive it's not
cancer. It's now Tuesday.

Steve and I walk out shakily, elated, relieved, and with the
old adrenaline pumping. It's time to cheer. We head over to one
of our favorite Japanese restaurants for a celebration dinner. At
this point in my life, I don't drink much. Ironically, for a couple of
years Steve has been giving me articles showing the link between
breast cancer and alcohol, and I have been cutting back. But
tonight I order a drink and rejoice. We have a lovely evening.
Still, there is just a little bitty scare underneath it all — what if the
doctor is wrong?

We wait for two days. Fortunately, my full schedule as a psy-
chotherapist distracts me. Then, Thursday afternoon, the phone
rings. Steve is home from work. I ask him to take the call, but I
stay to listen. He answers the phone. It's the doctor. Steve just lis-
tens for a minute or so and then says "Oh, no!" in much the same

---

*Currently, a breast biopsy is supposed to remove all of the tumor plus a vari-
able amount of the healthy tissue surrounding it. In other words, a lumpectomy
and breast biopsy can be one and the same. My surgeon, convinced that I didn't
have cancer, chose to remove only the tumor and no surrounding tissue (an excision biopsy). Therefore, I ultimately needed a second surgery.

tone my first husband said "Oh, my God!" when we were skidding off the mountain. I don't need to be told I have cancer.

That sinking feeling in the pit of my stomach is back, bigger and heavier than ever before. Shock hits me at full force. In this state of mind, I must decipher the meaning of my diagnosis.

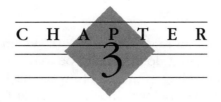

CHAPTER 3

Your Diagnosis

STEVE

If you're like most American women with breast cancer, you probably found the lump yourself. If you're under 40, the chances are you were told "let's follow it." Even if you're in your 40s, you may still have been given this advice. To comprehend why simply "following it" can be a mistake and before you decide what to do, you first need to understand how the doctor evaluates your risk.

PHYSICAL EXAM AND MEDICAL HISTORY

Most breast cancers are discovered as painless lumps. Many premenopausal women, however, have a condition that has commonly been called "fibrocystic disease" — painful breast lumps that change in the course of their menstrual cycle.* If a patient has both these symptoms and breast cancer, it may not be clear that the lump in question is painless.

If your sister has breast cancer or your mother had breast cancer before the age of 40 your risk is approximately

---

*Until recently, "fibrocystic disease" was considered an acceptable diagnosis for a variety of benign breast conditions. Currently, scientists are realizing that these conditions are not all the same, making the "garbage pail" diagnosis of fibrocystic disease increasingly unacceptable. As used in the remainder of this chapter, however, "fibrocystic disease" refers not to a specific medical condition but rather to the symptoms women have come to associate with this term; the term is still in widespread use and for our purposes the constellation of benign conditions it indicates may be considered together.

doubled.[1] It now appears that prostate cancer in male relatives may also raise your risk. Nonetheless, such a history can only increase your suspicion if you find a lump — it doesn't diagnose anything. In fact, more than 90 percent of women with breast cancer are the first in their family to ever get the disease.

The textbooks tell us that breast cancer may be "fixed" in place; yet, when first discovered, most breast lumps, including cancerous ones, are generally movable.

Textbooks also tell us that breast cancer may be associated with dimpling of the skin or recent retraction of the nipple, yet most of the time these signs are *not* present when the cancer is first discovered.

Breast cancers are described as "stony hard" in textbooks. If the lump is small and relatively deep in the breast, "stony hard" may be easier to talk about than to feel.

Confused? So should your doctor be. Determining how suspicious a lump is by simply feeling it is often difficult. Whenever the lump isn't *clearly* linked with "fibrocystic" changes, it's imperative that you don't just "follow it." You need to do something.

What do we mean by "fibrocystic" changes? We mean a lump in a premenopausal woman that a doctor determines is definitely painful, movable, changeable in the course of the month, not hard, and not associated with skin dimpling or nipple retraction. If that picture isn't clear to both you and your doctor, the lump should be considered suspicious. If you're postmenopausal, *any* breast lump should be considered suspicious.

Why do doctors so frequently tell women (particularly younger women) "let's follow it"? Perhaps it's because, statistically, the vast majority of lumps in premenopausal women are fibroadenomas (benign tumors) or conditions formerly considered "fibrocystic disease." The younger the woman, the greater the chance that the lump is not cancer. You, however, are not a statistic. If you are the uncommon 35-year-old with breast cancer, who cares what the diagnosis is in most other women?

From Discovery of a Lump to Diagnosis

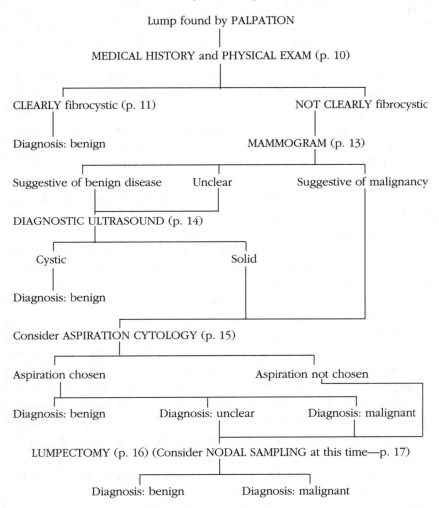

Lump found by PALPATION

MEDICAL HISTORY and PHYSICAL EXAM (p. 10)

CLEARLY fibrocystic (p. 11)   NOT CLEARLY fibrocystic

Diagnosis: benign   MAMMOGRAM (p. 13)

Suggestive of benign disease   Unclear   Suggestive of malignancy

DIAGNOSTIC ULTRASOUND (p. 14)

Cystic   Solid

Diagnosis: benign

Consider ASPIRATION CYTOLOGY (p. 15)

Aspiration chosen   Aspiration not chosen

Diagnosis: benign   Diagnosis: unclear   Diagnosis: malignant

LUMPECTOMY (p. 16) (Consider NODAL SAMPLING at this time—p. 17)

Diagnosis: benign   Diagnosis: malignant

Even if you're postmenopausal, many lumps turn out to be benign. These lumps are usually painless and don't show any cyclical changes. Therefore it's often easy for the doctor to be confused.

The punch line? If you and your doctors aren't 99 percent sure of the diagnosis, don't let them "follow it" — do something!

MAMMOGRAPHY

Before we get to the diagnosis of a lump you've already felt, let's talk for a moment about *screening mammography.* "Screening" implies the mammogram is done when there is no palpable lump nor anything else indicating cancer. Until recently, most medical groups in the United States have recommended a screening mammogram by age 40.[2] The American Cancer Society still does, but the National Cancer Institute has stopped advocating routine mammograms for women between the ages of 40 and 50. In 1994, editorials in the *Journal of the American Medical Association*[3] and the *American Journal of Public Health*[4] recommended against routine screening in this age group. In the rest of the world, screening mammograms are typically not recommended until age 50.[5] A combined analysis of the best research finds it completely useless in younger women,[6] despite a few studies suggesting the opposite.[7] One recent study found that more than half of the breast cancers investigated were not detectable by mammography in premenopausal women.[8]

Why the issue of age? The younger the woman, the denser her breast tissue. The denser the breast, the more difficult it may be to see the lump on a mammogram. The dense tissue makes screening mammography less useful in younger women.

Virtually all doctors acknowledge that screening mammograms are useful for women age 50 or older. Even in older women, however, screening mammograms can be a two-edged sword. For each life saved that results from early cancer detection due to a screening mammogram, many women will have unnecessary biopsies as a result of a suspicious mammographic finding. I believe that until the research is more definitive, screening mammograms should not ordinarily begin before age 50. My position is shared by the Task Force on Periodic Health Examinations (Canada), Canadian Workshop Group, U.S. Preventive Service Task Force, American College of Physicians, International Union Against Cancer, and the European Group for Breast Cancer Screening.[9]

It's important to distinguish between *screening* versus other mammograms. A mammogram done to look at a specific lump is *not* a screening mammogram. Once a suspicious lump is found, a mammogram should be done even in younger women because it can sometimes help in the diagnosis.

If there is any suspicion about a lump, then the first step is usually mammography. If you find a suspicious lump and ask the doctor to order a mammogram, you'll probably get one. If your doctor won't order a mammogram, consider finding another doctor. The risk of the mammogram is slight because the amount of radiation exposure is quite small. Sometimes the mammogram will reveal telltale suggestions of cancer that won't be apparent from other diagnostic procedures. For example, certain patterns of calcium deposition, a potential sign of cancer, may show up clearly only on the mammogram.

Some mammograms are better than others. Make sure the equipment has been certified by the American College of Radiology, the person doing the mammogram is a mammography technician, and the films are being read by a certified radiologist.

If a mammogram shows something suspicious, the doctor will generally follow it with further diagnostic tests. If the mammogram doesn't show anything, but you have a questionable lump, shouldn't the doctor continue to push for a more definitive diagnosis anyway, particularly if you're premenopausal? Absolutely.

DIAGNOSTIC ULTRASOUND

Diagnostic ultrasound (which exposes you to no radiation) may be the next step unless the mammogram has already made the diagnosis relatively clear. Although diagnostic ultrasound can't help definitively diagnose cancer, it can reveal whether the lump is hollow ("cystic") or solid. Cancers and fibroadenomas are solid. Cysts are hollow and fluid-filled. If the lump is clearly hollow, you have nothing to worry about. If the lump is solid, it's still probably not cancer; but more investigation is necessary.

Many doctors skip ultrasound in their hunt for a diagnosis. This path may make sense if you're postmenopausal because, beyond the menopause, cysts are less likely. If you're pre-menopausal, however, I believe it's usually a mistake to skip this step. Ultrasound is noninvasive, safe, and relatively inexpensive; it requires little time and may provide very useful information. Calling ultrasound "enormously helpful," researchers at the Elizabeth Wende Breast Clinic of Rochester, New York, feel that it permits them to "cancel many unnecessary [surgical] biopsies."[10] Newer, high-resolution ultrasound is being developed that is expected to dramatically reduce the number of unnecessary biopsies done as a result of equivocal findings on mammograms.

BIOPSY

Assuming that breast cancer has not been ruled out on the basis of physical exam, medical history (questions about pain and the constancy or cyclic nature of the lump), mammography, and possibly ultrasound, the next diagnostic step — biopsy — usually tells you definitively whether or not you have cancer. You have a choice in how the biopsy is done, but your doctor may not tell you about all the options. You should be aware of all your choices and discuss them with your doctor.

Aspiration Cytology

The least invasive procedure used to make the diagnosis, aspiration cytology (also called aspiration biopsy or needle biopsy), is often done at this point in the diagnostic process. Just as frequently, however, it isn't even mentioned as an option. What is it, and why do some doctors choose to do it while others avoid it?

With aspiration cytology the first step is the administration of a local anesthetic. Then a needle is inserted into the tumor and some fluid and/or cells are removed. If clear fluid is removed and the "tumor" disappears, the diagnosis is usually very simple: it was just a cyst. (As noted earlier, you and the doctor may have already learned this much with the aid of the ultrasound.) On occasion, nothing can be withdrawn by the needle, in which case the aspiration is a waste of time and a surgical biopsy becomes necessary. In most cases, however, something can be extracted. Under a microscope, pathologists look for cancer cells that were removed by the aspiration. If they find such cells, the patient has breast cancer.

Now comes the rub — and the reason why some doctors shy away from using this simple, relatively noninvasive procedure. A doctor who is not very experienced with this technique may get a "false negative" result — that is, even though cancer cells are present, they aren't extracted through the needle. Therefore, the pathologist looking through the microscope doesn't find any evidence of cancer, and the pathology report is negative.

How can this happen? If the doctor improperly places the needle and therefore misses the actual tumor, cancer cells won't be extracted. How often does this happen? In experienced hands, accounts of as few as one mistake per seventy breast cancers have been reported.[11] Other studies, however, report missing 15 percent,[12] 23 percent,[13] or even more.

Should you opt for aspiration? If the medical doctor you're working with doesn't have a long and proven track record with the procedure, probably not. Otherwise, it's the least invasive, quickest, and most inexpensive way to diagnose breast cancer.

To review, a "positive" aspiration virtually proves that cancer does exist. The reliability of a "negative" report depends upon the track record of the medical physician doing the procedure. Discuss the option of aspiration with your medical doctor.

Lumpectomy

If aspiration is not done, if the mammogram suggests cancer, or if the results of these tests are unclear, the next step is surgical biopsy. A lumpectomy is the removal of the tumor plus a surrounding layer of healthy tissue. Apparently healthy tissue is removed to ensure that no cancer extends beyond the edges of the biopsy. If the surgeon removes only what appears to be the tumor, some cancer cells are often left in the body.

Occasionally surgeons who think they "know" the tumor is benign may suggest not taking this extra tissue. (Removing the lump without a margin of safety is sometimes referred to as an "excision biopsy" instead of lumpectomy.) I recommend against this, as does Bernard Fisher, M.D.,[14] probably America's foremost breast cancer researcher. The cosmetic benefit in not taking a little extra tissue is usually minor. The hassle and anxiety of a second surgery may be major.

Lumpectomy has an additional benefit. If cancer is diagnosed, lumpectomy is usually the only breast surgery necessary; therefore, it can act not only as a means of diagnosis but also as the primary surgical treatment — all in one step.

Don't be afraid to ask questions before having this procedure done. If your doctor talks in medical gobbledygook, ask him or her to define terms. There is no reason you shouldn't understand thoroughly what's going on. All important terms can be explained in everyday language. Don't be afraid to take another few minutes of the doctor's "precious time"; what's happening is too important, and for whom is time more precious than you?

AXILLARY DISSECTION/NODAL SAMPLING

There is at least one more testing decision to be made. When a lumpectomy is done or shortly thereafter, the surgeon will want to "sample" lymph nodes or "dissect the axilla" (armpit). Your surgeon probably won't ask whether you want the sampling done. Nevertheless, you may choose not to have it done.

Breast cancer typically spreads first to lymph nodes in the axilla on the same side as the affected breast. Surgical removal of a few of these nodes ("sampling") or a total clearing of the lower parts or all of the axillary nodes ("partial or total axillary dissection") is generally done as a matter of course. If cancer has spread to nodes, the typical prognosis is worse than if the nodes are cancer-free, but still much better than if cancer has spread to an unrelated organ of the body. In other words, women who find they have "nodal involvement" or "positive nodes" frequently still live a full life span.

Why do nodal surgery? To begin with, if the nodes are not examined, you and the doctor won't know what "stage" the cancer is in — that is, how far it has spread. Without this information, you and your surgeon won't know your prognosis (theoretical chances of survival). Remember, however, that *theoretical* chances of survival may have very little to do with what actually happens to you. The situation is somewhat analogous to betting on horses; knowing the odds doesn't tell you who's going to win.

Although most medical doctors would disagree, I believe that your physician's knowledge of your prognosis may not be important. Do you really want to have this additional surgery to satisfy the doctor's curiosity or to "further science?" Remember, your body belongs to you — not to your doctor.

But nodal sampling will also give *you* the prognosis. If this information is important to you, go for it. If you feel that getting more bad news might interfere with your mental state and, therefore, your ability to fight the disease, consider this issue before agreeing to lymph node surgery. Only you should decide whether you want or need this prognostic information.

What are the chances that your nodes are positive? If there are hard swellings in the involved armpit, the chance is very high. Otherwise, it's a real crap shoot. On average, about half of all breast cancer patients are initially diagnosed with "positive" nodes (meaning that cancer has spread to the axilla) and about half have "negative" nodes. The smaller the size of the breast tumor, the lower the chances that there is nodal involvement. However, even with very small tumors (1 centimeter or 0.4 inches), nodal involvement is not rare.

Nodal sampling is also done to determine drug treatment. But, as we see in Chapters 7 and 9, regardless of nodal status, *postmenopausal* women are often offered tamoxifen (a drug with fewer side effects than chemotherapy) instead of chemotherapy. Most researchers believe chemo provides little additional benefit after menopause. Even those who disagree frequently don't use nodal status to determine whether chemo should be given to a postmenopausal woman.[15]

If you are *premenopausal,* nodal status can play an important role in determining drug treatment. As we see in Chapter 7, although the side effects and risks of chemotherapy may be high, there is a clear benefit for premenopausal women with positive nodes in using chemo; the size of the benefit is much smaller for those with negative nodes.

If you are considering whether to sample nodes, read Chapters 7 and 8 and talk with your doctor before making a decision. If you decide to use chemo regardless of your nodal status, there may be no need to sample nodes unless you want to know your prognosis. If you choose to avoid chemo regardless of your nodal status, it also may not make sense to have your nodes sampled except to satisfy your own curiosity.

Will surgically removing the nodes increase your chances of a cure? If the nodes turn out to be cancer-free, the answer is no. Even if cancer is found in the nodes, it is not at all clear that removal influences the outcome. Some studies suggest no effect, while others show 5–10 percent improvement in cure rates.[16] When nodal dissection does appear to improve survival,[17] it may simply be because it leads to other therapies. As far as many oncologists are concerned, nodal surgery is done primarily for diagnostic (not healing or curing) purposes. Citing the work of Bernard Fisher, the American Cancer Society's textbook reports, "as a therapeutic maneuver . . . routine axillary dissection has been shown not to improve survival."[18]

It is true that total nodal removal (called "nodal clearance") results in better "local control"; once found and totally removed, cancer in the axilla is less likely to reappear in that part of the body (compared with cancer in patients who have limited or no nodal sampling).[19] Whether this procedure extends life expectancy is not at all clear, however. In other words, researchers find it does not reduce the likelihood that cancer will return to the breast or the chance that cancer will appear in an unrelated part of the body. It is this appearance of cancer in an unrelated part of the body (called "distal metastasis") that is life-threatening. Sampling more versus fewer nodes is also associated with relatively better "local control," but also doesn't affect life expectancy.[20] While

some medical doctors say "obviously knowledge of the true axillary nodal status is mandatory,"[21] examination of the research generally shows no overall survival advantage, despite the apparent
common sense of finding and physically removing cancerous
nodes. It seems that cancer is not a local disease that goes away
by "killing it wherever you find it." It's much harder to understand
and treat than that. Although the average medical doctor may still
operate out of the old "find and destroy" model, the leaders at the
forefront of research have abandoned this approach because it just
doesn't fit with the facts that surround this elusive disease.[22]

Is there a downside to the nodal surgery? Of course — as
there is with all surgery. Residual pain, numbness, swelling
and/or weakness in the involved arm are possible consequences
that should be discussed ahead of time with your surgeon.

If you do decide to go ahead with one of the axillary procedures, don't agree to sampling.[23] Unlike partial or total dissection,
mere sampling is a hit-or-miss affair, sometimes falsely suggesting
that the nodes are "normal" when dissection would have proven
otherwise.

Because the issue of nodal surgery is complex, let's review
the information. Whether you have nodal surgery done should be
your choice. If cancer is diagnosed, the surgeon will automatically
assume nodal surgery will be done and will not offer you a
choice — you must ask for it. If nodal surgery is done, it should
be dissection, not sampling. There appear to be good reasons for
having your nodes examined: because you want to know your
prognosis or because you've decided to do chemo only if cancer
is found in the nodes. In addition, having all the axillary nodes
removed will reduce the chance that cancer will come back to
that specific region of the body (although such removal does not
appear to extend life).

BLOOD TESTS

You should know what each test means. Blood will be drawn and
a chem screen or SMAC 20 (the number may vary) and a CBC will
be run.

The Chem Screen (SMAC)

The chem (chemistry) screen provides much information. It's the human equivalent of having your car engine hooked up to a diagnostic computer when it's time for a tune-up. In addition to providing information about your risk of heart disease, diabetes, gout, and a wide variety of other conditions, it may reveal something about cancer. If liver and bone enzymes, analyzed as part of the chem screen, are elevated, they may suggest that the breast cancer has spread to these parts of the body. Today, most women do not have such advanced disease when diagnosed. Therefore, the chances are good that these indices will come back negative (normal). It should be mentioned that most liver and bone diseases not related to cancer can also elevate the enzymes in question. Therefore, an elevation does not necessarily indicate the spread of cancer.

The CBC

The CBC is a complete blood count. When advanced, cancer has a tendency to cause anemia. But anemia unrelated to cancer is very common, especially in premenopausal women. The anemia associated with iron deficiency is supposed to result in abnormally small blood cells, while the anemia of cancer (or other chronic diseases) is not supposed to change blood cell size. In reality, however, neither of these factors is inevitably true. If the cause of anemia is unclear to your doctor, simple and reliable tests can be done to rule out iron deficiency.

CHEST X RAYS

In addition to a chem screen and CBC, a "chest film" (X ray) will be ordered to see whether the cancer has spread to the lungs. As mentioned earlier, women today are usually diagnosed before distal metastasis (spread to an unrelated organ) occurs, and so the chest X ray will usually be normal.

PATHOLOGY REPORT

Pathologists are medical doctors who examine the surgically removed tissue, whether from an aspiration or lumpectomy. You'll
probably never meet these people. Although it's possible for their
work to be done while you're still on the operating table, for the
sake of the hospital's convenience and cost, the results are usually not available until several days after surgery. The report is
written in medical jargon and won't be intelligible. Nonetheless,
asking your physician about the following parts of the pathology
report will tell you a great deal more than just whether the tumor
was benign or malignant.

Tumor Size

Assuming the diagnosis is cancer, ask your doctor about the size
of the actual tumor — *not* the size of the entire lump that was removed. Unfortunately, although pathologists are supposed to report *both* sizes, they don't always do so. The actual cancer is generally smaller than the tissue that was removed. All talk about
"how big the cancer is" must refer to the tumor alone. Without
this information, the chance for an accurate prognosis is reduced.
If an ultrasound had been done previously, however, it will frequently show the size of the tumor itself.

    If the tumor is 1 centimeter or less, it is considered very
small. The chances are high that you'll live to a ripe old age without any further treatment. (Chapter 7 will review the data showing that chemotherapy may be superfluous for patients with no
nodal involvement and very small cancers.) Tumors between 1
and 2 centimeters are considered small. A tumor of 2 centimeters
or less, accompanied by no nodal involvement, is called "stage I"
— the most localized level of breast cancer. As we shall see in
other chapters, long-term studies show that 70 percent of stage I
patients are cured after conventional treatment.

    A moderate-sized tumor of 2 to 5 centimeters, if accompa-
nied by limited or no nodal involvement, is regarded as "stage II,"
as are smaller tumors if they are accompanied by limited nodal

involvement. Stage II is still considered early breast cancer. The chapters in this book that deal with treatment are written for women with stage I or II disease. Treatments for later-stage disease are not directly addressed in this book.

Histopathology

If your tumor is diagnosed as cancer, the pathologist will indicate what type it is — the "histopathology." By far the most common type of breast cancer is "infiltrating ductal carcinoma." When doctors speak about breast cancer, the information they provide usually refers to this form. "Infiltrating lobular carcinoma" behaves approximately the same way. Some of the less common types (particularly *in situ* carcinomas) are not as likely to metastasize (spread to a distant part of the body) and therefore carry unusually good prognoses. There may be less justification for using radiation or chemotherapy with such breast cancers. Therefore, ask the surgeon what "histopathologic type" your breast cancer is and the meaning of that information.

Grade

The pathologist is also routinely supposed to report the grade of the tumor, though sometimes this isn't done. "Very well differentiated" (often called "low grade" or "grade 1") indicates that the cancer cells have an orderly distinct appearance relatively similar to normal cells when viewed under the microscope. Such a designation is associated with a lower chance that the cancer will ever spread compared with "poorly differentiated" (also called "high grade" or sometimes "grade 3") cancers. Therefore, particularly when lymph nodes are cancer-free, a low-grade tumor reduces the justification for chemotherapy.

A separate grade is given to the centers (nuclei) of the cancer cells; this is called "nuclear grade." The grade and/or nuclear grade are generally on three-point scales. (Note: If you discuss the issue of grade, make sure your oncologist speaks in terms of "very well," "moderately well," or "poorly" differentiated rather than giving the grade a number. The numbering systems are not always consistent, especially for nuclear grade.) Don't be concerned if either grade is the middle ("moderately differentiated" or "grade 2") of the three possibilities. Few tumors are very well differentiated (some studies report less than one in ten) and mid-grade tumors are still considered a good sign.[24] How much "grade" tells us is still in debate; but it's my belief that, when studied more carefully, it will turn out to be an important factor.

Receptor Status

Pathology labs automatically run estrogen receptor tests on breast cancer cells. The cancer will be labeled "estrogen receptor positive" (ER-positive) or "negative." ER status is often important in determining treatment. For example, if you're postmenopausal and the tumor is ER-positive, tamoxifen, a non-chemo drug, is more likely to help you. Your ER status will be given an exact number, which may also prove useful to you in determining treatment approaches. For example, some premenopausal women with a high ER number are better candidates for ovarian removal than for chemotherapy (see Chapter 7).

Women with ER-positive status are considered to have a slightly better prognosis. Progesterone receptor status (PR) will also be reported. PR-positive is also thought to be a good sign. In terms of your prognosis, however, you shouldn't read too much into hormone receptor status. It has been found that many women (possibly 40 percent) with ER-positive status have defective receptors; these women may not have any survival advantage and would not necessarily be helped by tamoxifen.[25] Unfortunately, sorting out which receptors are functional and which aren't is something even your hospital is not yet capable of.

Ploidy Status

Many high-tech hospitals are now adding other tests, also done with tumor tissue. The tumor may be labeled as "diploid" or "aneuploid." Diploid indicates that the cancer cells have the normal number of chromosomes; aneuploid cells do not. Diploid tumors are associated with a better prognosis for some patients,[26,27,28] but it remains unclear how vital this factor may be; other components, such as tumor size, nodal status, and grade, are probably more important. Most women with breast cancer have aneuploid status; but, considering our limited understanding, such a finding should not be weighed very heavily.

S-Phase Fraction

The other new, frequently employed test using tumor tissue is called "SPF" or S-phase fraction. High SPF appears to indicate that the tumor cells are reproducing at a fast rate; of course, this is not a good sign. Some researchers consider SPF below 7 as low and above 12 as high.[29,]* Other researchers use 10 as a cutoff point between high and low SPF.[30] In some studies, a high SPF correlates with a worse prognosis,[31,32,33] while in others, it has made little or no difference.[34,35] Although a lower SPF is considered a good sign, we need to know more before attributing too much importance to it.

Sometimes ploidy status and SPF are combined into what is called the DNA index. If your pathology report lists a DNA index score instead of ploidy status and SPF, ask your doctor to explain the results to you.

Many other new prognostic markers associated with the pathology report are being developed, and it's possible that one or more of these may be included in your work-up. But there is not enough research yet about the tests not specifically mentioned here to tell us how reliable their results will prove to be.

---

*Each lab has its own ranges for high and low SPF; go with the criteria established by your lab.

SCANS

Your doctor may order bone and liver scans to evaluate the possibility that cancer has metastasized to these parts of the body. These studies should be done only if you have symptoms suggesting such a spread. Bone metastasis is usually suspected when there is bone pain. Liver metastasis may change the feel of your liver during the physical exam and, as mentioned above, will typically change your chem screen. If your history, physical, and chem screen are all normal, I believe it makes no sense to do routine scans because it's most unlikely that the scans will come up with new information. The relative uselessness of running routine bone scans has recently been reviewed in the *Journal of the American Medical Association*.[36] The researchers report that it takes more than 1,500 bone scans to find one case of bone metastasis if the patients have no symptoms. Most "positive" scans in asymptomatic women turn out to be false positives; in other words, they worry the woman for no reason. If the scan does accurately diagnose metastasis, the cancer is no longer curable. These tests are neither simple nor reasonably priced, so if your doctor has no special reason to suspect metastasis, consider carefully before agreeing to have the scans run.

THE NEW GENETIC TEST

By the time you read this, BRCA1, a gene causing breast cancers to be passed down in families, will probably have been isolated. Once it is, a blood test will soon follow allowing all women to know if they carry the gene. Those who do are thought to account for only 2 to 4 percent of all breast cancer. But if you have the disease, your sisters and daughters need to seriously consider the test because women carrying the gene have a lifetime risk for breast cancer of more than 85 percent. If your doctors are unfamiliar with BRCA1, they should start by reading the research.[37,38,39] If breast cancer is rampant in your family, more cumbersome (and soon to be obsolete) genetic testing is already available if multiple family members are willing to give blood samples.

QUESTIONS TO ASK YOUR DOCTOR AFTER A CANCER DIAGNOSIS

Following is a list of questions you need to ask and a review of what the answers indicate. See pages 291–2 for a copy of these questions with spaces for you to fill in your doctor's answers.

About the Chem Screen (SMAC)

Are my liver and bone enzymes normal?
> An answer of "yes" combined with no symptoms of liver or bone disease suggests that cancer has not spread to those organs. It also means that it's probably pointless to do bone or liver scans. An answer of "no" requires immediate attention and perhaps scans.

About the CBC (Complete Blood Count)

Is my CBC normal?
> An answer of "yes" merely confirms that you don't have the anemia of late-stage cancer. An answer of "you're anemic" usually just means iron deficiency, but have your doctor follow up with specific iron-deficiency tests.

About the Chest X Ray

Is my chest X ray normal?
> An answer of "yes" suggests that cancer has not spread to the lungs. Confirmed evidence of spread to the lungs means late-stage disease.

Pathology Report

When the pathology report becomes available to your doctor, you will be told if you have cancer. If you do, there are many relevant questions you should ask to help you determine your treatment plan.

How large was the cancer?
Make sure the doctor distinguishes your question from "how large was the tissue that was cut out?" See page 22 for an explanation of tumor sizes.

What kind of breast cancer is it?
"Infiltrating ductal" or "infiltrating lobular" are the two most common answers. If the reply is anything except these two, it's possible that your prognosis is exceptionally good. See page 23.

What grade is the cancer?
"Very well differentiated" or "highly differentiated" (also sometimes called "grade 1") is a good sign. "Moderately differentiated" ("grade 2") is not a bad sign. "Poorly differentiated" increases the likelihood that chemotherapy or ovarian ablation should be seriously considered. See Chapter 7.

Is my estrogen receptor status considered positive?
In general, an answer of "yes" is thought to improve prognosis somewhat. More specifically, if you are postmenopausal and your status is positive, the drug that you will probably be offered, tamoxifen, is more likely to help fight the cancer. See Chapter 9.

What is my specific estrogen receptor level?
For premenopausal women, the specific ER level may determine whether surgical removal of the ovaries might be more effective than chemotherapy. Such an approach may have fewer side effects. See Chapter 7.

Do I have diploidy?
An answer of "yes" is considered a good sign, but the importance of this test is still in debate.

Is my S-phase fraction relatively low?
An answer of "yes" means that the cancer cells were reproducing slowly — a good sign. Again, this test's importance is still unclear.

References

1. Colditz, G. A., et al. Family history, age, and risk of breast cancer. *JAMA* 1993;270:338–43.

2. Jenks, S. ACS keeps mammography guidelines for women under 50. *J Natl Cancer Inst* 1993;85:348–9.

3. Love, S. M. and D. L. Davis. Mammographic screening. *JAMA* 1994;271:152–3 [editorial].

4. Shapiro, S. The call for change in breast cancer screening guidelines. *Am J Publ Health* 1994;84:10–11 [editorial].

5. Vanchieri, C. Europeans say screen only women age 50 and older. *J Natl Cancer Inst* 1993;85:350.

6. Elwood, J. M., B. Cox, and A. K. Richardson. The effectiveness of breast cancer screening in young women. *Curr Clin Trials* 1993;2:227.

7. Nystrom, L., and L. Larsson. Breast cancer screening with mammography. *Lancet* 1993;341:1531–2.

8. Day, P. J., and G. E. O'Rourke. The diagnosis of breast cancer: a clinical and mammographic comparison. *Med J Astral* 1990;152:635–9.

9. Elwood, J. M., B. Cox, and A. K. Richardson. The effectiveness of breast cancer screening in young women. *Curr Clin Trials* 1993;2:227.

10. Logan-Young, W. W., et al. Letter. *N Engl J Med* 1993;328:811.

11. Dixon, J. M., et al. Fine needle aspiration of the breast: importance of the operator. *Lancet* 1983;ii:564 [letter].

12. Masood, S., et al. Prospective evaluation of radiologically directed fine-needle aspiration biopsy of nonpalpable breast lesions. *Cancer* 1990;66:1480–7.

13. Hindle, W. H., and J. Navin. Breast aspiration cytology: a neglected gynecologic procedure. *Am J Obstet Gynecol* 1983;146:482–7.

14. Fisher, B. Reappraisal of breast biopsy prompted by the use of lumpectomy. *JAMA* 1985;253(24):3585–8.

15. Fisher, B. A biological perspective of breast cancer: contributions of the National Surgical Adjuvant Breast and Bowel Project Clinical Trials. *CA* 1991;41(2):97–111.

16. Kinne, D. W. The surgical management of primary breast cancer. *CA* 1991;41(2):71–84 [review].

17. Cabanes, P. A., et al. Value of axillary dissection in addition to lumpectomy and radiotherapy in early breast cancer. *Lancet* 1992;339:1245–8.

18. Keys, H. M., R. F. Bakermeier, and E. D. Savlov. Breast cancer. In *Clinical oncology,* 6th ed., ed. P. Rubin, American Cancer Society, Rochester, NY, 1983.

19. Mattheiem, W., et al. Axillary dissection in breast cancer revisited. *European J Surg Oncol* 1989;15:490–5.

20. Benson, E. A., and J. Thorogood. The effect of surgical technique on local recurrence rates following mastectomy. *European J Surg Oncol* 1986; 12:267–71.

21. Kjaergaard, K., et al. Probability of false negative nodal staging in conjunction with partial axillary dissection in breast cancer. *Br J Surg* 1985;72:365–67.

22. Fisher, B. A biological perspective of breast cancer: contributions of the National Surgical Adjuvant Breast and Bowel Project Clinical Trials. *CA* 1991;41(2):97–111.

23. Kinne, D. W. The surgical management of primary breast cancer. *CA* 1991;41(2):71–84 [review].

24. Fisher, E. R., et al. Pathologic findings from the National Surgical Adjuvant Breast and Bowel Project (protocol 4). *Cancer* 1993;71:2141–50.

25. Benz, C. C. DNA binding estrogen receptor isoforms in breast cancer. American Cancer Society's Thirty-second Science Writers' Seminar, Daytona Beach, Florida, March 27, 1990.

26. Clark, G. M., et al. Prediction of relapse or survival in patients with node-negative breast cancer by DNA flow cytometry. *N Engl J Med* 1989; 320(10):627–33.

27. Joensuu, H., et al. DNA index and S-phase fraction and their combination as prognostic factors in operable ductal carcinoma. *Cancer* 1990;66:331–40.

28. Beerman, H., et al. DNA flow cytometry in the prognosis of node-negative breast cancer. *N Engl J Med* 1989;321(7):473–4 (letter).

29. Sigurdsson, H., et al. Indicators of prognosis in node-negative breast cancer. *N Engl J Med* 1990;322(15):1045–53.

30. Stol, O., et al. S-phase fraction is a prognostic factor in stage I breast carcinoma. *J Clin Oncol* 1993;11:1717–22.

31. Joensuu, H., et al. DNA index and S-phase fraction and their combination as prognostic factors in operable ductal carcinoma. *Cancer* 1990;66:331–40.

32. Sigurdsson, H., et al. Indicators of prognosis in node-negative breast cancer. *N Engl J Med* 1990;322(15):1045–53.

33. Stol, O., et al. S-phase fraction is a prognostic factor in stage I breast carcinoma. *J Clin Oncol* 1993;11:1717–22.

34. Clark, G. M., et al. Prediction of relapse or survival in patients with node-negative breast cancer by DNA flow cytometry. *N Engl J Med* 1989; 320(10):627–33.

35. Kute, T. E., et al. The use of flow cytometry for the prognosis of stage II adjuvant treated breast cancer patients. *Cancer* 1990;66:1810–6.

36. Schapira, D. V., and N. Urban. A minimalist policy for breast cancer surveillance. *JAMA* 1991;265(3):380–2 [review].

37. Breo, D. L. Altered fates — counseling families with inherited breast cancer. *JAMA* 1993;269:2017–2022.

38. King, M. C., et al. Inherited breast and ovarian cancer — what are the risks? What are the choices? *JAMA* 1993;269:1975–80.

39. Biesecker, B. B., et al. Genetic counseling for families with inherited susceptibility to breast and ovarian cancer. *JAMA* 1993;269:1970–4.

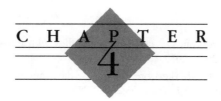

My Reaction to Diagnosis

CATHY

After getting the news I had the "the big C," I was overwhelmed by a confusion of feelings — many of them contradictory. Everything seemed blurred; it was hard to say exactly what I felt. My first thought was, "This is too much for us to bear alone. We need our friends." Three of our closest friends arrived within an hour. We stayed up late, going through the initial shock together. There were tears and even a little laughter. No one held back. The experience was incredible and just what I needed. Before this I had often dealt with painful feelings by turning inward, always with self-destructive results. This time I made a different choice.

Looking back now, I see this decision as pivotal; by bringing friends in at the beginning, I had support and understanding right away. Paradoxically, I was starting to take charge of my life at the very point it was seemingly spinning out of control. There were many emotional upheavals down the road, but I would not be facing them alone.

There were eight days between the diagnosis and my surgery. I tottered between hope and despair. One moment I was confused and uncertain about what to do; the next, I would be full of treatment ideas: laugh therapy, counseling, Hoxsey formula, vitamins, surgery. Then back to feeling alone and unsupported . . . then I would feel truly supported . . . then guilty for feeling alone and unsupported . . . next, a moment of peace . . . then angry, angry, angry with nothing to focus my anger on . . . then angry at myself for being angry and fatalistic because I thought this attitude would kill me for sure . . . then depressed as I realized the focus of my days for the foreseeable future was going to be cancer and more cancer.

During this week I had my first panic attack. I woke up at 3 A.M. from a bad dream about cancer. I was so filled with fear that I couldn't get enough air. I felt totally alone, though Steve was sleeping beside me. When I started to cry, he woke up, and we held each other. I talked about how scared I was until I finally calmed down and could breathe again.

In the course of one week, I reviewed the research with Steve, had my first visit with the naturopathic doctor who would guide my treatment, scheduled surgery for a lumpectomy, went in for a second opinion, had my first counseling appointment to deal with the overwhelming feelings, started reading Bernie Siegel's *Love, Medicine, and Miracles,* and called family and friends with the news. Through all this turmoil, I continued to see my clients.

Calling my parents was agonizing. While I needed their support, I knew the situation would cause us all pain. I knew they'd try their best to support me. When my mother asked what she could do, I suggested she call Karen, my sister, and John, my brother. I told her I'd contact my youngest brother, Mark. I knew these calls would be very difficult for Mom, but I needed her to make them for me. I waited a day to call Mark, to avoid phoning on his birthday and having my diagnosis irrevocably associated with it.

When I called my friends Blaze and Bob in southern California, I had to tell their machine, "it's an emergency, please call as soon as possible." Bob relayed the message to Blaze when she called him up to check in while bringing her students home from a tournament. She called me from the same pay phone at the freeway rest stop. I felt that I had dropped a huge burden on her, but I needed her. Full of love, she was ready to skip school to be with me at once, despite her dedication to teaching. Instead, we decided she'd come to Portland in a week.

We called other friends near and far. Steve made many of the calls and then told me what people said. I wanted my friends to know what had happened so that they would understand if I wasn't up to business as usual; I valued the love they expressed through Steve and their understanding that I was too overwhelmed to respond personally.

I sought support also by reading a book about cancer written for patients, but doing so was tough. The book aroused overpowering emotions. So I read in bits and pieces, digesting what I could.

Reviewing the research was another complicated experience. Research articles are as impersonal, cold, and unemotional as you can get. I trudged through dry data about this or that type of chemotherapy and mortality rates in the three-year prospective study versus the five-year retrospective study. The researchers write as if these numbers don't represent people, real people who lived and died.

And then there is that lovely word *remission*. People aren't ever cured of cancer; they're just "in remission." For me, before my surgery, remission meant it was just a matter of time before IT came back. IT was always lurking there ready for its encore performance.

Trying to process this research in the middle of my emotional turmoil was tough. More often than not, I had to ask Steve to read and explain the meaning of the various research articles. Was the research "good"? How big was the sample? How long was the follow-up? How was the study set up? What was all that gobbledygook in the conclusion supposed to mean? Why don't researchers use plain English? I was thankful that Steve could translate the most complicated medicalese into a simple word that anyone could understand, but I raged at the writers, wondering why they couldn't be so straightforward.

As I read, questions nagged at me: What does the research say compared with what the medical doctor said about radiation, chemotherapy, and surgery? Whom should I trust when the research and the doctor conflict?

Getting a second opinion helped a little. The medical doctor was compassionate and not defensive about alternative medicine — a pleasant surprise. He treated me warmly and concurred with the surgeon that I should go ahead with the lumpectomy. He understood my reluctance regarding chemotherapy and radiation. Although I left the appointment comforted, my anxiety continued to increase as I moved inexorably toward surgery, still questioning what to do about nodal sampling, radiation, and chemotherapy.

I also visited a counselor. Fortunately, one I respected could see me promptly. I have been through a fair amount of therapy in my adult life — individual, couple, and group. For the most part I have found it to be healing and productive, but also scary and painful. I knew that difficult feelings would surface: fear, anger, hopelessness, and despair. Intellectually, I knew they needed to be faced, but I feared they might compromise my immune system. So I felt anxious at my first appointment. With the therapist, I explored my fear and sense of isolation. Discussing my feelings allowed me to feel compassion for myself. After one session I felt stable for the first time since the nightmare began. We agreed to meet weekly.

That I continued to see my own clients surprised many people. Though it was hard to psych myself up for work each day, it turned out to be therapeutic. For the hours I saw clients, I could put my problems aside. I immersed myself totally in my clients' issues. I chose not to tell them about my diagnosis until much later. Continuing to lead my "normal" life gave me hope.

Looking back now at these experiences, I'm amazed how quickly I mobilized. At the time, though, I felt as if my feet were in concrete, I had no voice of my own, and Steve had to take care of me. And at the beginning of this nightmare, I was very dependent on him. While that dependence made me feel small and powerless, it also helped me feel less alone.

But a few days after the diagnosis, Steve told me he couldn't be my doctor or make my decisions for me. He said he would support me 100 percent whether I chose conventional or alternative treatments, or a combination; but if he chose for me, it might create great difficulties for both of us.

Intellectually, I knew he was right. He had to be my husband, not my doctor. Emotionally, however, I felt abandoned, which only exacerbated my feelings of being totally alone.

Only the cancer patient knows the loneliness of waking up and realizing, every day, "Oh, my God, it wasn't just a bad dream." I've read many personal accounts by cancer patients and I invariably think, "Yes, that's just what I felt." Loneliness and fear seem to be universal for those of us who've had cancer, but communicating these feelings to those who haven't feels impossible. This truth does not discount the pain and alarm that Steve, my friends, and my family suffered. Their experience is simply different. I know, because I've been in that spot too. My mother-in-law, whom I loved very much, died of cancer — years before my diagnosis.

No matter how much love and support are received, the person who gets the diagnosis still feels completely alone with this terrible potential thing called death.

Treatment Choices

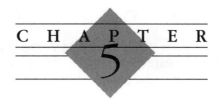

C H A P T E R

5

Your Surgical and Radiation Choices

STEVE

In the late nineteenth century, conventional medicine decided that breast cancer was a localized disease: It started in the breast, spread to lymph nodes, and finally went to other parts of the body. A leading proponent of this theory was William Halsted, an American surgeon. He believed that surgery was unsuccessful because not enough tissue was being removed, which left cancer cells in the vicinity of the breast. These cells then spread, ultimately causing fatal metastases. The solution, according to Halsted, was to cut out more tissue, thus advancing ahead of the cancer. His surgery included removal of chest muscles in addition to the breast and accompanying lymph nodes. The removal of muscle led to gross mutilation to the chest wall and shoulder, as well as decreased strength and increased swelling in the attached arm.

It has been said in reference to Halsted's procedure that "Aggressiveness is often a sign of desperation, and surgical aggression is no exception."[1] By 1888, concerns were being voiced about the lack of supporting evidence for radical surgery.[2] Halsted's results, published shortly after,[3] did little to allay those apprehensions. In fact, many of the patients he termed "successes" were followed for only a few months after their surgeries. Today, such a report would be considered meaningless. Years after the original report, many researchers proved Halsted wrong.[4] Breast cancer could not be sliced into submission by excessive surgery. Nevertheless, despite a lack of scientific support, the Halsted radical mastectomy became conventional medicine's treatment of choice and remained so until recently.* A pessimistic review of the Halsted failure appeared more than 30 years ago in the *Journal of the American Medical Association*,[5] but it went unnoticed by most surgeons.

Increasingly in the 1970s and 1980s, research from Italy and America compared the Halsted radical mastectomy to less invasive surgery. In 1985, the *New England Journal of Medicine* published the results of a National Adjuvant Breast and Bowel Project (NSABP) study that followed patients for ten years.[6] Patients who had their chest muscles spared did no worse than those given the Halsted radical.

The NSABP is perhaps America's most esteemed breast cancer research group, and the *New England Journal of Medicine* the most respected conventional medical journal. Finally, the tide had turned. Today, virtually all surgeons and oncologists agree that the Halsted radical has little place in the treatment of breast cancer.

According to current conventional medical thinking, Halsted miscalculated because "micrometastasis" — the early traveling of a few cells to other parts of the body — usually occurs *before* breast cancer is diagnosed. Current theory suggests that even radical surgery is usually too late to be curative by itself. But if surgeons really believe that breast surgery is usually "too late," why do they always do it? And how does this new hypothesis explain the good health of the many women who are disease-free thirty years after diagnosis? Many of these women have been treated only with surgery. Proponents of the theory claim that surgery must have *preceded* micrometastases for these lucky women. Such an explanation doesn't prove the theory — it simply helps to justify it.

Its proponents suggest that the new micrometastasis theory is quite different from Halsted's thinking. But in reality, it's only a minor modification — and almost as poorly supported by science. To this day, no one really understands breast cancer. Given two women with the same initial level of disease, doctors don't know

---

*Mastectomy means surgical removal of the breast. In discussing this procedure with your doctors, note that the pronunciation follows the spelling: mastectomy.

why one survives and the other doesn't. Proper treatment would be based on a clear understanding of the disease — something we still lack. I doubt we'll get much closer to the truth until we look at factors seemingly removed from the breast — like the immune system, the mind, and other ways in which the body defends itself against cancer. Lacking such fundamental understanding, *no one really knows how to treat breast cancer.*

It's uncomfortable for both patients and doctors to admit this. It's easier to create theories that camouflage our ignorance and then sugar-coat them to "protect" women from the anxiety of the truth. Yet, by acknowledging our lack of understanding, we can look at surgical and other options (both conventional and alternative) without the distortions of unsupported hypotheses.

TOWARD MORE LIMITED SURGERY

Removal of the breast ("simple mastectomy"), combined with removal of lymph nodes, replaced Halsted's radical mastectomy. The new procedure is called a "modified radical." It is now well accepted that this less-mutilating surgery offers the same chance of cure as did the Halsted radical. As discussed in Chapter 3, removal of lymph nodes is done primarily for diagnostic, not curative purposes. Therefore, the "simple mastectomy" alone is the therapeutic equivalent of the Halsted radical.

Many years before the modified radical came into vogue, a courageous American surgeon, George Crile, Jr., began experimenting with even less invasive surgery.[7] He reported surprisingly good results with simple removal of the lump — what we now call lumpectomy.[8] Later, researchers from Milan, Italy, studied women with tumors less than 2 centimeters (0.8 inches) who did not clearly have cancer in their lymph nodes. The Milan group reported that removing lymph nodes and doing "quadrantectomy" (removal of a quarter of the breast surrounding the tumor) plus radiating the breast achieved the same results as the Halsted radical.[9] They concluded "mastectomy appears to involve unnecessary mutilation. . . ."

In studies comparing various surgical treatments after five years[10] and again after eight,[11] the NSABP reported that the chance of survival was the same regardless of whether patients had lumpectomy alone, lumpectomy with radiation, or mastectomy. This finding was surprising because when only limited surgery is done (lumpectomy), the addition of radiation is generally considered mandatory in order to duplicate the cure rate achieved with mastectomy.

The NSABP eight-year follow-up focused on comparing lumpectomy alone to lumpectomy plus radiation. Though survival was the same in both groups, the chance that cancer would return locally to the breast increased dramatically when radiation was omitted. After eight years, only one woman in ten had had a local recurrence in the breast after lumpectomy with radiation. But four women in ten had had a local return of cancer *without* the radiation.

Reports followed from other research centers with corroborating evidence. The chance of survival was the same regardless of the surgery. However, when lumpectomy was done *without radiation,* there was a high risk of a "local recurrence" in the breast. From these studies, the currently accepted surgical choices became (and remain) lumpectomy plus radiation or mastectomy (usually done as a modified radical including removal of lymph nodes). If you have early-stage breast cancer you probably were or will be given these choices, though there are several occasions where only mastectomy is offered.

The primary reason for choosing lumpectomy over mastectomy is cosmetic — the breast is saved. But if the tumor is large and the breast is small, conserving the remainder of the breast may not achieve any cosmetic purpose. In such cases a lumpectomy loses its advantage. Also, if the breast has more than one tumor, two lumpectomies may also result in an unsatisfactory appearance.

Some surgeons are afraid to do lumpectomy with a relatively large tumor even when (due to the position of the tumor or the size of the breast) the cosmetic outcome will be good. Such a position appears to lack scientific support. Lumpectomy is as effective as mastectomy with tumors at least as large as four centimeters.[12] Therefore, tumor size should probably not rule out lumpectomy.

Lumpectomy is generally accompanied by radiation (see the section, "Radiation Versus No Radiation," later in this chapter). Radiation should not be used in patients who have had previous breast irradiation or who have severe lung disease. In such cases, mastectomy may be the only surgical choice offered.

If you are not being offered lumpectomy, ask why. If you're uncomfortable with the answer, consider getting a second opinion. The majority of early-stage breast cancer patients should be given a choice.

MASTECTOMY VERSUS LUMPECTOMY

If you're given the choice, why even consider mastectomy? Why cut more when cutting less has the same result? There are several reasons. Some of them make sense, but others don't.

When the whole breast is removed, you can avoid radiation. Radiation requires almost daily office visits for about five or six weeks. Terminal cancer patients frequently receive radiation treatments (often to reduce bone pain) from the same doctors. So spending time in the radiation therapist's waiting room may make you feel as if you're visiting the morgue; it won't bring your spirits up.

There are other reasons to consider avoiding radiation. Occasionally, radiation will damage a rib or a lung, or even increase the risk of heart disease.[13] In some cases, radiation has damaged nerves that supply the hand or arm, leading to pain and loss of function.[14] It may also scar or discolor the breast or reduce your energy level for months. The skin over the breast may thicken. Modern radiation techniques limit most of the exposure to just the breast — decreasing, but not eliminating, these risks.

Radiation is, in itself, carcinogenic — though the number of cancers caused by breast radiation appears to be small. Increases in cancer in the opposite breast have been reported to be negligible[15] except for women younger than 45.[16] The younger you are when radiation is done, the more likely it is to eventually cause another cancer. Lung cancer risk doubled in patients treated with radiation during the 1970s and early 1980s,[17] but current radiation techniques should reduce this risk. Nonetheless, current and past smokers already at high risk of getting lung cancer should be concerned about breast radiation.

For some women, surgical and radiation decisions *appear* to be clear: If you want to preserve the breast, do lumpectomy and radiation. If you're most worried about the potential side effects of radiation or you don't have time for radiation, mastectomy is the right choice. Unfortunately, for many women, the choice is not that simple.

Many women choose mastectomy to "get the cancer out of my body for good." If you can't shake this feeling, you may need the mastectomy for psychological reasons. Be aware, however, that following surgery, women who choose mastectomy have no less fear of a recurrence than do women who choose lumpectomy.[18]

Before you choose to have a mastectomy out of fear, I believe it's important for you to understand the facts. Having a mastectomy to "make sure they got it all" is a decision not grounded in reality. Remember — the chance of long-term survival is the same whether you choose mastectomy or lumpectomy. Moreover, when radiation is added to the lumpectomy, the chance of a local recurrence is also the same. In fact, if your chief concern is to stay alive, there's at least one reason *not* to choose mastectomy.

If a local recurrence happens after mastectomy, it occurs on the chest wall. A chest wall recurrence is an ominous sign — much harder to treat than a typical recurrence in the breast following lumpectomy. So, although removing the breast does not reduce your risk of anything except potential radiation side effects, it probably does put you at greater risk should you have a local recurrence.

Unfortunately, the fear that underlies the desire to "just get it out of my body for good" is not always alleviated by the surgeon. To this day, it's not uncommon to hear male surgeons (particularly those who were educated before the end of the Halsted era) say "if you were my wife, I'd tell you to just get rid of it."

The chance that this unscientific advice will be offered to you by the surgeon varies widely depending upon where you live and who your surgeon is. States requiring doctors to tell patients about surgical options have fewer mastectomies and more lumpectomies than do other states.[19] Regional differences also exist, with higher levels of mastectomy in the South and lower levels in the Northeast. A breast cancer patient age 65 to 79 in Massachusetts is six times more likely to have a lumpectomy than is her sister in Kentucky.[20] This variance has nothing to do with science and a lot to do with medical philosophy. Younger, urban, better educated, more affluent women are more likely to choose lumpectomy.[21] It's not because their cancers are different from their older, poorer, country cousins. It's just more likely that they're better informed.

THE VALUE OF SURGERY

Researchers now all agree: the chance of survival is the same regardless of whether you choose lumpectomy or a mastectomy. But a question begins to emerge when different treatments result in the same rate of "cure": how much better are they than no treatment at all? In other words, does surgery really save the lives of breast cancer patients?

Breast cancer death rates have not improved in the last half century, which suggests that all conventional approaches should at least be questioned — even surgery. It has been many years since any group has gone without treatment. Instead, surgical patients have been compared with breast cancer patients who received no treatment in the nineteenth and early twentieth centuries.[22] But these untreated women were almost all late-stage and, by definition, not representative of early-stage patients. To compare modern surgical results in early-stage patients with the rapid deaths reported many years ago in untreated late-stage patients is inappropriate. A recent review of cancer surgery concluded that "the reason for the lack of evidence for surgery's efficacy might be that it is not effective. . . ."[23] A respected scientist once said "there is no provable concept that treatment has altered the course of the disease."[24]

Despite our lack of proof, however, it's most likely that surgery does increase cure rates. At least for women over 50, routine screening mammography is associated with better survival (see Chapter 3). Surely getting a mammogram does not reduce the chance of dying. It must be the conventional treatment that follows early diagnosis. And because the only constant in conventional treatment is some form of surgery, we can assume that surgery helps. I find this logic compelling.

Even here, an independent analysis of the original screening/mortality data (done by a skeptic of surgery) found that women who accepted mammography screening (and later had a lower risk of dying from breast cancer) were quite different from those who refused to get mammograms.[25] The women who agreed to mammographic screening not only had a lower death rate from breast cancer, but they also had a lower death rate from everything else! They were simply a different group of women. Nonetheless, consistent reports that early screening (followed by surgical treatment) leads to a lower risk of dying from breast cancer strongly suggests that surgery helps your chances.

Virtually all conventional medical doctors believe surgery to be essential. I have talked with many alternative practitioners who have treated and observed breast cancer using a variety of techniques over the years, and all but one believe that surgery increases cure rates. Choose which surgery suits you, but make a choice and act on it.

WHEN SHOULD SURGERY BE DONE?

Most breast cancers are not fast-growing malignancies. Nonetheless, most doctors (of all kinds) agree that postponing surgery for weeks or months can do no good and might result in a reduced chance of cure.

For postmenopausal women, no more need be said. But for premenopausal women, some researchers have come to believe that the point in the menstrual cycle at which the surgery is done may strongly influence the likelihood of a recurrence.

In 1989, William Hrushesky reported that patients who underwent surgery at or near the time of their periods had a much higher risk of recurrence and death than did women whose surgery was done at other times.[26] Other researchers looked for this relationship but found that surgical timing did not make any difference.[27,28]

For a while, the subject died. But then researchers from Guy's Hospital in London reported that timing of surgery made a dramatic difference.[29] There was just one problem — the "safe" and "dangerous" times of the month did not correspond with those previously reported by Hrushesky.

At least one paper has subsequently supported the Guy's Hospital findings[30] but others have not.[31–35] An analysis that compares a dozen studies looking for a relationship between timing of surgery and long-term outcome has found no consistency.[36] Yet Hruschesky and Guy's Hospital both continue to claim that timing is important.[37,38]

If we look for a common thread weaving together the reports that find that surgical timing counts, days 18–20 of the menstrual cycle appear to be a particularly good time to have surgery. The lack of consistency in the research, however, makes it difficult to know the value of such specialized timing. If you are premenopausal and your surgery is planned near days 18 through 20 of your cycle, you might want to play it safe and try to move it to one of these dates if possible.

Discuss this issue with your surgeon. Every surgeon should have easy access to the research cited in this section — it all comes from major medical journals. Although it's too early to know whether timing is important, I'm disturbed by the large differences in recurrence and death rates reported in those few studies which actually claim that timing counts.

BREAST RECONSTRUCTION

Following a mastectomy, surgical reconstruction is possible. So the one advantage of lumpectomy — good cosmetics — may also be obtained by many mastectomy patients. But, depending upon how it's done, reconstruction can be relatively major surgery and may require more than one operation. Moreover, while implants do not cause cancer,[39] they have been linked to other serious problems.

An implant can impair the ability of doctors to read future mammograms.[40] The rupture of an implant requires its removal, but sometimes the rupture doesn't cause symptoms. The consequence of a "silent" rupture remains controversial. A slew of unanswered questions about safety eventually led the FDA to pull silicon implants from the breast augmentation market, though they are still available to breast cancer patients.[41]

Silicon implants are associated with a wide variety of poorly defined symptoms. They may mimic rheumatoid arthritis, chronic fatigue syndrome, lupus erythematosus, systemic sclerosis, or other serious diseases.[42]

Migration of silicon from the implant into areas of inflammation has been documented,[43] suggesting that escaping silicon may have caused the inflammation. Of 33 women complaining of joint symptoms after breast implant surgery, 24 improved within two years after the implants were removed, according to researchers at the University of South Florida College of Medicine.[44]

Frequently, the body will try to surround the implant — a condition called spherical contracture. As a result, the breast feels excessively hard, and the implant may look more like a grapefruit and less like a natural breast. According to a recent *New England Journal of Medicine* article, contracture has been reported in 38 percent of those receiving implants for reconstruction following mammography.[45] Some contractures are barely noticeable, but others require removal of the implant.

Except for contracture, most side effects appear to be uncommon, though the reconstructed breast will never have the same sensation as a normal breast. To put implant-related side effects in context, Marcia Angell, a doctor and an editor of the *New England Journal of Medicine,* tells us that more than nine out of ten women receiving silicon implants have been satisfied with the results.[46]

Reconstruction can take place without a silicon implant. The most common substitute involves complex surgery where skin and muscle from the back or abdomen is used to form the reconstruction. These procedures avoid the need for silicon but leave scars on the back or abdomen, may cause abdominal or back muscle weakness, and require a longer hospital stay and as much as ten hours of surgery. Before any reconstructive surgery, talk with the surgeon. Ask to see "after" pictures not just of the surgeon's best work, but of a variety of patients.

Another option, dramatized by the recent *New York Times Magazine* cover showing a former model with her mastectomy, is to choose not to have reconstructive surgery. While many women will be self-conscious without reconstruction or prostheses, some are more uncomfortable covering up what has happened. Not everyone wants to yield to the pressure of trying to look "good." The important thing is to make the right choice for you — not what might be the right choice for other women.

RADIATION VERSUS NO RADIATION

"What is the medical logic for substituting useless and unnecessary radiation for useless and unnecessary surgery?"[47] So said Irwin Bross from Roswell Park Memorial Institute, a leading cancer treatment center in Buffalo, New York. Yet virtually all women who choose lumpectomy will be told they must do radiation. Somewhere between these two disparate positions lies the truth. A review of the facts may leave you agreeing that radiation is necessary for most lumpectomy patients. But if you wish to avoid radiation, read on — it's not *always* mandatory.

Recall that radiation does not alter your chance of surviving breast cancer. On the other hand, radiation does significantly reduce the risk that cancer will return locally to the breast. Local recurrences in the breast are treatable and generally not fatal;* nonetheless, having a breast cancer recurrence is at least a cause of enormous anxiety.

If you choose lumpectomy and your chance of local recurrence is high, it's clearly best to do radiation. The question, then, is who is at high risk and who is not?

---

*What kills patients is the spread of cancer to distant parts of the body — distal metastasis. And distal metastasis is not affected by radiating the breast.

Other researchers from Roswell Park reported that lymph node involvement does not increase the risk that breast cancer *returns locally to the breast*.[48] Therefore, having positive nodes doesn't automatically mean radiation must always accompany lumpectomy.

However, the same researchers did find two factors that predicted the chance of local recurrence: age and tumor size. Twenty women who had tumors less than 1 centimeter in size were followed for four years. None had a local recurrence *despite the fact that all the women had only lumpectomy and no radiation.* "The incidence of recurrence was directly correlated to the increasing size of the tumor. . . ." These findings suggest that women with very small tumors may be good candidates for considering lumpectomy without radiation.

The Roswell Park Researchers also followed thirty-one women over 70 years of age. Only one had a local recurrence *even though they had only lumpectomy and no radiation.* The recurrence rate for women in their 30s, on the other hand, was 40 percent. This underscores the need for very young women to include radiation if they opt for lumpectomy.

The benefits of radiation for different age groups following limited (quadrantectomy) surgery was explored by the Milan group mentioned earlier.[49] They studied patients with tumors smaller than 2.5 centimeters. When patients of all ages were considered together, the local recurrence rate after 39 months was almost zero in the group receiving radiation and 8.8 percent without it. But the women who were over 55 years and didn't have radiation had a local recurrence rate of only 3.8 percent — again revealing that older women may not always need radiation. The local recurrence rate for women under 55 without radiation was over 15 percent during the same period.

Canadian researchers from Princess Margaret Hospital in Toronto followed 1,504 patients for 26 years.[50] One-fourth had lumpectomy without radiation, suffering a local recurrence rate of 29 percent, compared with 14 percent for those who had radiation. Most of the local relapses occurred in the first three years. Those women who did have a local recurrence in the breast lived for an average of almost nine years *after the relapse*. (Remember, a local relapse after lumpectomy is not nearly as serious as a chest wall relapse after mastectomy.) As expected, radiation did not affect survival. Also, in keeping with other research, younger women (in this case, under 46 years old) had a greater risk of relapse than did women 46 or older.* Although a relationship between tumor size and the chance of local recurrence wasn't initially apparent, a follow-up report found a higher risk for women with tumors over 2 centimeters.[51] The second report also found that "poor nuclear grade" (see Chapter 3) significantly increased the risk that cancer would return locally to the breast.

These Canadian researchers looked for a subset of patients who were at very low risk of a local recurrence despite having lumpectomy without radiation. But no matter how they defined their patients (on the basis of tumor size, age, etc.), no group achieved a 95 percent chance of avoiding local recurrence unless they also had radiation. As a result, the Princess Margaret Hospital researchers recommended that "all patients receive breast irradiation."[52]

But researchers at the Royal Marsden Hospital in London came to the opposite conclusion. They followed node-negative women treated with quadrantectomy but no radiation for five to fourteen years. All had tumors less than 2 centimeters in size. The researchers concluded, "routine postoperative radiotherapy can be safely omitted in certain cases."[53] Again, younger women had a high risk. Only 10 percent of the postmenopausal group had suffered a local recurrence within five years, with almost no local recurrences beyond the first five years. But 24 percent of the small group of premenopausal women had had a recurrence during that same time. Women under 46 had a 36 percent chance of recurrence; those who were older had half that risk.

Swedish researchers have studied lumpectomy with and without radiation in node-negative women with tumors of 2

---

*Dividing women into groups who are under or over 46 is a result of research design — not physical considerations that separate women at this particular age.

centimeters or less.[54] After five years, almost nine out of ten patients without radiation had not suffered a local recurrence. As expected, with radiation, the recurrence rate was even lower, but survival was the same.

Researchers from the University of California at San Francisco studied lumpectomy without radiation regardless of nodal status or tumor size.[55] Because women with large tumors were not excluded, without radiation, the overall local recurrence rate was high. After two years, 19 percent of the lumpectomy-only group had already suffered a local recurrence. When very small (1 centimeter or less) tumors were excluded, the recurrence rate jumped to 28 percent after only two years. But when the removed lump had no microscopic trace of cancer on its outer edge (meaning that all the tumor was removed), only three of thirty-two women had had a recurrence. Other researchers agree with this finding — when cancer cells are left in the breast due to inadequate surgery, the risk of local recurrence goes up.[56]

If you have concerns about radiation side effects, have a very small tumor, and/or are beyond your mid-40s, you may still be considering lumpectomy without radiation. Before making a decision, review this checklist and then talk with your doctors. Without radiation:

- The overall risk of local recurrence increases sharply.
- The chance of long-term survival remains unaffected.
- Tumors of 1 cm or less have a low risk of local recurrence.
- Women in their 30s have a high risk of local recurrence.
- Women in their early 40s have a relatively high risk of local recurrence.
- Women in their 70s or older have a low risk of local recurrence.
- There is an increased chance of local recurrence for women with tumors of high nuclear grade (see Chapter 3).
- It's particularly important that the lumpectomy removes all cancer cells in the vicinity ("microscopically clean margins"), or local recurrence is likely.

Before making a decision about mastectomy, lumpectomy, radiation, or reconstruction, also be sure to read *Dr. Susan Love's Breast Book,** which clarifies these procedures, supplying answers that can be provided only by a breast surgeon.

References
1. Skrabanek, P. False premises and false promises of breast cancer screening. *Lancet* 1985;ii:316–9 [review].
2. Jackson, A. On carcinoma of the breast and its treatment. *Med Press* 1888;i:552–3.
3. Halsted, W. S. The results of operations for the cure of cancer of the breast performed at the Johns Hopkins hospital from June 1889 to January 1894. *Johns Hopkins Hosp Rep* 1894;4:297–356.
4. Skrabanek, P. False premises and false promises of breast cancer screening. *Lancet* 1985;ii:316–9 [review].
5. Lewison, E. F. An appraisal of long-term results in surgical treatment of breast cancer. *JAMA* 1963;186:975–8.
6. Fisher, B., et al. Ten-year results of a randomized clinical trial comparing radical mastectomy and total mastectomy with or without radiation. *N Engl J Med* 1985;312:674–81.
7. Crile, G. Jr. Results of simplified treatment of breast cancer. *Surg Gynecol Obstet* 1964;118:517–23.
8. Crile, G. Jr. Management of breast cancer: limited mastectomy. *JAMA* 1974;230:95–8.
9. Veronesi, U., et al. Comparing radical mastectomy with quadrantectomy, axillary dissection and radiotherapy in patients with small cancers of the breast. *N Engl J Med* 1981;305:6–11.
10. Fisher, B., et al. Five-year results of a randomized clinical trial comparing total mastectomy and segmental mastectomy with or without radiation in the treatment of breast cancer. *N Engl J Med* 1985;312:665–73.
11. Fisher, B., et al. Eight-year results of a randomized clinical trial comparing total mastectomy and lumpectomy with or without irradiation in the treatment of breast cancer. *N Engl J Med* 1989;320:822–8.
12. Habibollahi, F., and I. S. Fentiman. Breast conservation techniques for early breast cancer. *Cancer Treat Rev* 1989;16:177–91 [review].

Dr. Susan Love's Breast Book (Addison-Wesley, Reading, Mass., 1990) is available in both hardback and paperback at most bookstores.

13. Haybittle, J. L., et al. Postoperative radiotherapy and late mortality: evidence from the cancer research campaign trial for early breast cancer. *BMJ* 1989;298:1611–4.

14. Sikora K. Enraged about radiotherapy. *BMJ* 1994;308:188–9.

15. Storm, H. H., et al. Adjuvant radiotherapy and risk of contralateral breast cancer. *J Natl Cancer Inst* 1992;84:1245–50.

16. Boice, J. D. Jr., et al. Cancer in the contralateral breast after radiotherapy for breast cancer. *N Engl J Med* 1992;326:781–5.

17. Neugut, A. K., et al. Lung cancer after radiation therapy for breast cancer. *Cancer* 1993;71:3054–7.

18. Lasry, J-CM., and R. G. Margolese. Fear of recurrence, breast-conserving surgery, and the trade-off hypothesis. *Cancer* 1992;69:2111–5.

19. Ganz, P. A. Treatment options for breast cancer — beyond survival. *N Engl J Med* 1992;326:1146–8 [editorial].

20. Nattinger, A. B., et al. Geographic variation in the use of breast-conserving treatment for breast cancer. *N Engl J Med* 1992;326:1102–7.

21. Lazovich, D. A., et al. Underutilization of breast-conserving surgery and radiation therapy among women with stage I or II breast cancer. *JAMA* 1991;266:3433–8.

22. Bloom, H. J. G. The natural history of untreated breast cancer. *Ann NY Acad Sci* 1964;114:747–54.

23. Benjamin, D. J. The efficacy of surgical treatment of cancer. *Med Hypothesis* 1993;40:129–38.

24. Jones, H. Demographic consideration of the cancer problem. *Transactions N Y Acad Sci* 1956;18:298–333.

25. Fox, M. S. On the diagnosis and treatment of breast cancer. *JAMA* 1979;241:489–94.

26. Hrushesky, W. J. M., et al. Menstrual influence on surgical cure of breast cancer. *Lancet* 1989;ii:949–52.

27. Powles, T. R., et al. Menstrual effect on surgical cure of breast cancer. *Lancet* 1989;ii:1343–4 [letter].

28. Gelber, R. D., and A. Goldhirsch. Letter. *Lancet* 1989;ii:1344.

29. Badwe, R. A., et al. Timing of surgery during menstrual cycle and survival of premenopausal women with operable breast cancer. *Lancet* 1991; 337:1261–6.

30. Senie, R. T., et al. Timing of breast cancer excision during the menstrual cycle influences duration of disease-free survival. *Ann Intern Med* 1991: 337–42.

31. Low, S. C., M. H. Galea, and R. W. Blamey. Timing breast cancer surgery. *Lancet* 1991;338:691 [letter].

32. Goldhirsch, A., et al. Letter. *Lancet* 1991;338:691–2.

33. Sainsbury, R., et al. Timing of surgery for breast cancer and menstrual cycle. *Lancet* 1991;338:392 [letter].

34. Powles, T. J., et al. Timing of surgery in breast cancer. *Lancet* 1991; 337:1603–4 [letter].

35. Gnant, M. F. X., et al. Breast cancer and timing of surgery during menstrual cycle. A 5-year analysis of 385 pre-menopausal women. *Int J Cancer* 1992;52:707–12.

36. McGuire, W. L., S. Hilsenbeck, and G. M. Clark. Optimal mastectomy timing. *J Natl Cancer Inst* 1992;84:346–8.

37. Bluming, A. Z., and W. J. M. Hrushesky. Optimal timing of initial breast cancer surgery. *Ann Intern Med* 1992;268 [letter].

38. Gregory, W. M., et al. Letter. *Ann Intern Med* 1992;116:268–9.

39. Berkel, H., D. C. Birdsell, and H. Jenkins. Breast augmentation: a risk factor for breast cancer? *N Engl J Med* 1993;326:1649–53.

40. Handel, N., et al. Facts affecting mammographic visualization of the breast after augmentation mammaplasty. *JAMA* 1992;268:1913–7.

41. Kessler, D. A. The basis of the FDA's decision on breast implants. *N Engl J Med* 1992;326:1713–5.

42. Gard, Z. R., and E. J. Brown. Silicone breast implants and immunological disease. *Townsend Letter for Doctors* June,1993, pp.570, 572–3 [review].

43. Silver, R. M., et al. Demonstration of silicon in sites of connective-tissue disease in patients with silicon-gel breast implants. *Arch Dermatol* 1993;129:63–8.

44. Vasey, F. B., M. J. Seleznick, and B. F. Germain. The breast-implant controversy. *N Engl J Med* 1993;328:732–3 [letter].

45. Fisher, J. C. The silicon controversy — when will science prevail? *N Engl J Med* 1992;326:1696–8.

46. Angell, M. Breast implants — protection or paternalism? *N Engl J Med* 1992;326:1695–6 [editorial].

47. Bross, I. D. J. Radical mastectomy vs. quadrantectomy, axillary dissection, and radiotherapy for breast cancer. *N Engl J Med* 1981;305:1283 [letter].

48. Nemoto, T., et al. Factors affecting recurrence in lumpectomy without irradiation for breast cancer. *Cancer* 1991;67:2079–82.

49. Veronesi, U., et al. Radiotherapy after breast-preserving surgery in women with localized cancer of the breast. *N Engl J Med* 1993;328:1587–91.

50. Clark, R. M., et al. Breast cancer — experiences with conservation therapy. *Am J Clin Oncol* 1987;10:461–8.

51. Clark, R. M., et al. Randomized clinical trial to assess the effectiveness of breast irradiation following lumpectomy and axillary dissection for node-negative breast cancer. *J Natl Cancer Inst* 1992;84:683–9.

52. Clark, R. M., et al. Randomized clinical trial to assess the effectiveness of breast irradiation following lumpectomy and axillary dissection for node-negative breast cancer. *J Natl Cancer Inst* 1992;84:683–9.

53. Greening, W. P., et al. Quadrantic excision and axillary node dissection without radiation therapy: the long-term results of a selective policy in the treatment of stage I breast cancer. *European J Surg Oncolog* 1988;14:221–5.

54. Uppsala-Orebro breast cancer study group. Sector resection with or without postoperative radiotherapy for stage I breast cancer: a randomized trial. *J Natl Cancer Inst* 1990;82:277–82.

55. Lagios, M. D., et al. Segmental mastectomy without radiotherapy. *Cancer* 1983;52:2173–9.

56. Ghossein, N. A., et al. Importance of adequate surgical excision prior to radiotherapy in the local control of breast cancer in patients treated conservatively. *Arch Sur* 1992;127:411–5.

My Surgical and Radiation Decisions

CATHY

I was frantic. In the midst of suddenly discovering I might well be dead soon and, in the meantime, hacked apart, fried, or worse, I was supposed to decide everything. Immediately.

My surgeon gave me a "simple" choice: lumpectomy with radiation or mastectomy. He told me some women preferred a mastectomy. Weeks of radiation would then be avoided, along with its side effects. I'd just "get it over" in one fell swoop.

Sure. Just get your breast cut off and it's all over. Permit me to doubt. I'm rather attached to my breasts — downright fond of them. They're a part of my identity as a woman and an important part of my sexual pleasure. And breast cancer is a systemic disease anyway. Lopping off a breast doesn't necessarily mean it's "all over."

The tumor was small, so the cosmetic result of a lumpectomy would probably be good. Of course, lumpectomy would also be less invasive than mastectomy. The surgeon admitted that cutting more does absolutely nothing to improve survival chances. I chose lumpectomy.

Lumpectomy and radiation were offered as a package deal. Even though I felt pressured by the surgeon to have radiation treatments, I was against it, concerned about the side effects. The younger you are at the time of radiation, the more likely it is that radiation itself will eventually cause another cancer, though this risk is small. Agreeing to a treatment that was in itself potentially carcinogenic seemed ludicrous. I was only 43. The research also mentions that radiation can cause hardening and discoloration of the breast, as well as loss of breast sensitivity — not life-threatening issues, but ones that might have reduced my self-esteem and sexual enjoyment. Radiation can crack ribs or damage lungs. Additionally, the surgeon explained, radiation treatments can be psychologically trying. In the waiting room, I'd be surrounded by dying people, a situation that could be demoralizing. I knew that depression could affect the immune system, and I wanted to avoid any situations that might cause it.

Fortunately, Steve's search of the medical literature on radiation gave me the information I wasn't getting elsewhere. Radiation had been presented to me as a way to increase survival, but the research shows radiation does not increase life expectancy. It decreases only the incidence of local recurrence (see Chapter 5).

For many women, reducing the risk of a local recurrence is reason enough to undergo radiation. For me, it wasn't. Steve and I confronted my surgeon. He admitted radiation hadn't extended life "yet," as though he had reason to believe it would. In prescribing for me, the surgeon had introduced his personal beliefs as scientific truth. I had a right to know the difference.

Even my naturopathic doctor initially thought I should consider radiation. He studied the pathology report, looking for evidence of cancer in blood and lymphatic vessels. There wasn't any. He also checked to see if cancer had extended to the edge of the tissue that had been removed. It hadn't. He knew the tumor was small and low-grade. Only when he saw that all these indicators pointed toward a low risk of recurrence in the breast did he begin to support my choice.

I struggled to make the "right decisions" when every option had pros and cons and when no choice guaranteed perfect health. However, having made the decision to have a lumpectomy and not to have radiation was a relief. I felt I'd made the best choices I could with the information then available. Years later, I still feel that way.

However, there was still a surgical choice to be made, another part of the lumpectomy-radiation "package" — nodal dissection. The surgeon and Steve couldn't feel anything abnormal

under my arm. Given the small size of the breast tumor (1.1 centimeters), the lack of anything palpable meant I probably had
clean nodes. But "probably" still left about a 20 percent chance
that the cancer had already spread.

Nodal dissection was presented as something that must be
done with lumpectomy. Only my questions and Steve's research
of the medical literature made it clear that nodal dissection was
diagnostic, not therapeutic. It wouldn't buy me an extra day.

If any of my nodes contained cancer, the surgeon would
have recommended chemotherapy. I had already decided against
chemo (see Chapter 8). I knew there might be side effects from
the nodal surgery (see Chapter 3). And, I'd had enough bad
news. If I had cancer in my nodes, I didn't want to know.

You might want to know your nodal status and therefore
choose this surgery for that reason alone. Or you might well want
this information to decide about chemotherapy (or even ovarian
surgery). But if you can live without that knowledge, if you have
already decided about chemo, or are choosing tamoxifen instead
of chemo, you may want to avoid this surgery with its possible
side effects and extra expense.

Having decided on lumpectomy without radiation or nodal
surgery, I had to choose between hospital and day surgery. I
don't like hospitals, so that decision was easy.

Before the surgery, the surgeon led me to believe that the
shape of my breast would change very little. When I took the
bandages off for my first shower and looked down, I was aghast
at what appeared to be a big crater. I huddled in the tub, sobbing
uncontrollably. A few honest words from the surgeon would have
prepared me better for reality.

Neither did he warn me about the possibility of nipple sensitivity following surgery. In my case, this condition persisted for
months as nerve fibers regrew. It hurt, and I was frightened. I
thought something had gone horribly wrong with the surgery.
Again, preparation would have helped.

Now, five years after my surgery, the pain is gone, the scar
has faded, and the "crater" seems more like a deep dimple. In fact,
it just reminds me to count my blessings and be glad I'm alive.

In retrospect, I opted for the riskiest choice regarding the chance of a local recurrence. But the treatments I avoided wouldn't have added to my life expectancy. My choices leave me the lowest chance of treatment-induced side effects. My choices may well not be yours.

Yet, any choice is ultimately a gamble. I know I don't have a crystal ball, but I do have a sense of my own priorities. You do too. After you've read this book and listened to your doctors, it's still your body and your life.

CHAPTER 7

Should You Have Chemotherapy or Ovarian Ablation?

STEVE

For some people, improving their chance of survival, even marginally, is more important than anything else. Some feel this way even when they discover that most breast cancer patients obtain absolutely no benefit from chemotherapy, yet all patients suffer the side effects.

If you are trying to make a decision about chemo, you may be reading this chapter to gather facts.* If you'll endure anything to improve your chances just a wee bit, there's little point in reading further. Some breast cancer patients in virtually every group studied — pre- or postmenopausal, estrogen receptor (ER)-negative or positive, node-negative or positive, early stage or late stage — have shown at least marginal benefits from chemotherapy in several studies. (ER status is discussed in Chapters 3 and 9, and nodal status is discussed in Chapter 3.)

Note: If you're postmenopausal, your oncologist may be offering tamoxifen instead of chemotherapy because the former is less toxic and achieves similar results. If so, you may want to skip to Chapter 9. Regardless of your menopausal status, if it's clear to your oncologist that your chance of a recurrence is very low, you may not be offered chemotherapy and may choose to skip this chapter.

*For premenopausal women who wish to avoid chemotherapy, a conventional alternative, ovarian ablation, is discussed in this chapter.

Many medical doctors assume that a woman will take great risks in hopes of achieving such benefits. Remarks like the following are not uncommon: "Patients are willing to accept toxic treatment in exchange for quite modest gains in overall survival. . . ."[1] Although this quote may describe how the theoretical "average patient" feels, in real life there is no average patient. And you may not be willing to accept the risk of severe toxicity in exchange for "modest gains" that won't necessarily be yours anyway.

In making your chemotherapy decisions, you may seek answers to the following questions:

- What are the possible toxicities and how frequently do they occur?
- How likely is chemotherapy to help *me* — given my nodal, ER, and menopausal status?
- Do I have any therapeutically equivalent treatment options?

No doubt, your oncologist is familiar with much of what I'll say here. Oncologists administer advice based on their feelings about potential risks and benefits. They may have decided in advance what risk-to-benefit ratio they believe is appropriate for you. This chapter allows you to participate in that decision, instead of passively accepting the oncologist's opinion. As you read, take good notes. Write down questions that pop up, and ask your oncologist for answers.

Some oncologists won't take offense if you wish to make the ultimate decision about chemotherapy. Depending upon your situation, they may not want to shoulder all the responsibility when the best course is often unclear. Other oncologists may take your questions as an affront. But, remember, you have no obligation to accept such a response. Getting a second opinion has become an established procedure. If you're not being included in the decision-making process and want to be, consider seeing someone else.

THE CONCEPT OF ADJUVANT CHEMOTHERAPY

Adjuvant means "assisting" or "aiding." When a woman has early-stage breast cancer, surgery and sometimes radiation are the primary conventional therapies. They are used in hopes of removing or destroying the cancer. After these treatments, the patient may well be cured. If chemo is added several weeks following surgery, it's usually done as an adjunct — just in case.

Doctors use the term *adjuvant chemotherapy* to distinguish the use of chemo in early-stage cancer from the way chemotherapy is employed in late-stage disease. In advanced (or late-stage) disease, when cancer has spread to a distant part of the body, surgery and radiation are no longer curative and therefore may not even be used. Chemotherapy then becomes the primary treatment, used not to increase the chance of a cure after surgery and radiation, but by itself — and only to buy time.

If adjuvant chemo is added to early-stage treatment "just in case," the obvious question is, Just in case what? The current theory of breast cancer tells us that some women have "micrometastases" — tiny pockets of cancer that cannot be detected and might be knocked out with chemo. We don't know ahead of time who has these micrometastases. Therefore, the theory goes, most breast cancer patients should receive chemo unless it's quite clear they are at very low risk of a recurrence. In this way, the micrometastases will be destroyed before they can cause trouble.

In the last two decades, this new theory has swept through conventional medical thinking. In discussing the effects this recent theory has had on treatment, breast cancer patient and advocate Rose Kushner has said, "by the end of 1981 I sensed that indiscriminate, automatic adjuvant chemotherapy was replacing the Halsted radical mastectomy as therapeutic overkill in the United States."[2]

In Chapter 5, I discussed the Halsted radical mastectomy, which resulted from the theory that cancer starts in the breast and continues to grow from that point. It followed that the more flesh surgeons removed, the better the chance they had "gotten it all." Though this theory was never proved, the Halsted radical dominated medical treatment of breast cancer for most of this century. Now that the Halsted theory has been disproved, there is much less invasive surgery.

Virtually all medical doctors now realize that the spreading of cancer is not simply an extension of the breast tumor; they now accept that breast cancer is a "systemic disease," one that affects the whole body — a claim made by alternative doctors for decades. In reality, though, the conventional medical paradigm still doesn't treat breast cancer as systemic; it continues to view the disease as a group of microscopic, localized problems. Systemic theories do exist that focus on the body's own ability to fight the cancer, but such ideas have been only poorly explored and are not as yet taken seriously by conventional medicine.

The frequent existence of micrometastasis has been proven. Yet concluding that chemotherapy is the only or best way to deal with these pockets of cancer (or that the micrometastases will necessarily turn into life-threatening cancer) is still speculative. In a sense, we can say that this approach stands on about as much solid ground as did the old Halsted radical mastectomy theory.

The rush to add chemotherapy to the treatment plans of more and more breast cancer patients is of concern to some medical doctors. Michael Baum from King's College School of Medicine and Dentistry in London says drily, "overall, the results of chemotherapy have not been spectacular." Baum says that in order to make chemo look more impressive than it really is, researchers employ "strategies of torturing your data until it confesses."[3]

In 1992, an editorial in the *New England Journal of Medicine* claimed the new chemo studies at best "reflect a variable and, in most if not all cases, transient prolongation of survival for patients who would have died earlier without the treatment."[4] It goes on to say that most early-stage patients are cured by mastectomy or lumpectomy plus radiation alone. Obviously, these patients cannot benefit from chemo (having already been cured), but they will experience the toxicity. Among those not cured, "some would live a few months longer as a result of adjuvant therapy but would still die within the first decade after diagnosis. . . . A very few might gain decades of life as a result of treatment."

Despite these concerns, there is little question that chemo increases the chances of survival for some women. Doctors agree that we need to find better ways to identify these women. You may not agree with their interim prescription: "Until then we shall have to continue with our blunderbuss approach that treats all patients with toxic and expensive drugs to obtain marginal therapeutic benefits."[5]

THE CONCEPT OF "SUCCESS" WITH CHEMOTHERAPY

To evaluate the effects of chemotherapy, most research trials look at survival and disease-free survival — that's all. ("Survival" tells us how many people are alive and includes both those who are disease-free and those who have suffered a recurrence but remain alive.) Very few studies factor in quality of life. Most women have impaired quality of life from taking chemotherapy but relatively few benefit. The scale should weigh toxicity along with potential gains.

Why don't the oncologists who write the research consider quality of life? Rose Kushner says, "Most of the time, oncologists do not even see their patients during regular . . . appointments. In the United States, baldness, nausea and vomiting, diarrhea, clogged veins, financial problems, broken marriages, disturbed children, loss of libido, loss of self-esteem, and body image are nurses' turf."[6] Nurses don't publish studies of chemotherapy trials. Kushner goes on to describe Australian research showing that oncologists view side effects differently than patients do. The doctors tend to discount or be unaware of the extent of their patients' suffering.

While ignoring quality of life, most studies also seem relatively unconcerned with the amount of improvement resulting from chemotherapy as long as there is at least some statistically significant improvement. Frequently the improvement (measured by the proportion of women who actually benefited) is quite small. This fact is not sufficiently emphasized. If chemo were harmless, we wouldn't need large benefits before suggesting that these drugs be used. Because of substantial toxicity, however, researchers should be held to a higher standard before doctors begin to prescribe. The benefit should be more than just statistically significant before women are told to take these drugs.

Fortunately, some researchers have voiced concerns about the size of benefits in relation to toxicity. Authors of the National Surgical Adjuvant Breast and Bowel Project (NSABP) study defined the issue clearly:

> Does an improvement of 10 percent . . . justify the administration of therapy to an entire population [of node negative patients] when about 70 percent will survive free of disease . . . without [chemo] and about 20 percent will not benefit from [it]? . . . There are no criteria for making such a decision; it must be a value judgement.[7]

As a result of high toxicity and low therapeutic effect, Thomas Nealon Jr., professor of surgery at New York University School of Medicine, says, "The treatment of this tumor now has slipped from too much surgery to too much adjuvant therapy."[8]

When evaluating chemotherapy, we need to consider another issue. In most studies, disease-free survival improves much more than does life span (overall survival). At first glance, this makes no sense. If the patient is kept cancer-free for a longer period of time, she should live longer. The apparent contradiction may be explained in two ways. While chemo reduces the chance of a recurrence in the breast and lymph nodes, it does not appear to decrease the chance that a recurrence will take place in bone, liver, or lung.[9] And it's the recurrence of cancer in these distant parts of the body that is most likely to prove fatal. Some evidence suggests that the use of chemotherapy leads to a shorter survival time if the cancer does recur. A group of Japanese researchers has found that life span after recurrence is shortened by chemotherapy because patients previously treated respond poorly to subsequent chemo.[10] These researchers suggest that drug resistance may have developed. In other words, chemo may not work well if it is used twice. Patients treated with chemo the first time may stave off a recurrence longer than do untreated women, but they die faster after the recurrence. Thus the life expectancy for women treated with chemo twice may be about the same as that for women treated only upon recurrence. Here's one way to look at these statistics: If you are going to be one of the majority of early-stage patients whose cancer will not recur, why take chemotherapy? If you turn out to be one of those whose cancer will recur, why not consider saving chemo for a time when its potential benefits are most clearly needed?

Yet, these are not rhetorical questions. You don't know ahead of time whether a recurrence will happen. And some women are spared a recurrence by chemo. The best way to make the difficult decision to have or not to have chemotherapy is to arm yourself with information.

THE DRUGS

This section includes some graphic descriptions of chemotherapy toxicity. If you feel unprepared to read through it, just skip to "Chemotherapy and Node-Negative Women" (page 73) or "Chemotherapy, Ovarian Oblation, and Node-Positive Women" (page 82).

Most commonly, early-stage breast cancer patients are treated with a standard combination of chemotherapy drugs — cyclophosphamide, methotrexate, and fluorouracil. This combination is called CMF, the acronym deriving from the first letter of each drug. Some of the CMF story is relatively clear:

- CMF works better than any single drug.
- CMF administered over a six-month period is most effective. Therefore, you should not take CMF for more than six months.
- Starting CMF within a few weeks after surgery appears to be optimum.

Sometimes, adriamycin, prednisone, or several other drugs are used in combination with CMF (or instead of the cyclophosphamide) in treating early-stage patients. As yet, not enough is known about the relative merits of these other combinations compared with CMF. Because of this lack of information and because CMF (or a variant) is what early-stage patients are most commonly offered, I'll confine my comments to CMF. Before considering the pluses and minuses of this combination, let's look at each drug separately.

Cyclophosphamide

Cyclophosphamide is also known by its trade name, Cytoxan. "Cyto" refers to cells. "Tox" you don't need translated. Cytoxan evolved from mustard gas used to kill soldiers in World War I. It belongs to a group of chemotherapy drugs called alkylating agents, which are all considered extremely toxic.

Cyclophosphamide works by killing cells as they replicate. Patients taking cyclophosphamide feel sick because it does not selectively go after cancer cells; the human body is made up of cells that need to replicate. Therefore, the drug affects the whole body.

As a result, cyclophosphamide can be poisonous. It causes birth defects, so pregnant women can't take it. It appears in human milk, so women can't breastfeed when taking the drug.

Nausea and vomiting are common side effects, occurring in approximately 25 percent or 30 percent of patients on the drug. *Science News* quotes Thomas Burish, a psychologist at Vanderbilt University, as saying, "many patients come to dread chemotherapy so much that they vomit the night before treatment or in the waiting room."[11] It has been scientifically documented that just thinking about chemotherapy can induce nausea in patients familiar with its side effects.[12]

Cyclophosphamide frequently causes a cessation of the menstrual cycle in premenopausal women, a change that is often permanent. If menses do not return, the patient is sterile.

Because the reproduction of white blood cells (WBCs) is interfered with, the WBC count drops, sometimes dangerously. When the number of WBCs falls too low, the patient's immunity is impaired, rendering her susceptible to serious infection.

The drug also causes impaired wound healing. Hair loss occurs in about half the women taking cyclophosphamide. Although bleeding inflammation of the bladder is much less common, it can occur and be quite serious.

Though cyclophosphamide is used to treat cancer, it can also cause the disease — typically leukemia, lymphoma, or bladder cancer. The *New England Journal of Medicine* estimates that cyclophosphamide causes about one case of leukemia for every

2,000 women who take it.[13] Some researchers find higher risks with drugs of this type (alkylating agents),[14] while others don't report any increased risk.[15]

One in 2,000 is, of course, a very low risk considering that the drug is used to treat a life-threatening disease. Unfortunately, however, the leukemia doesn't necessarily occur in those who are most at risk of dying of breast cancer; it also affects those who are cured before the chemotherapy is administered.

Although most studies don't track it, fatigue is usually the most common side effect for breast cancer patients taking chemo, including cyclophosphamide. One study which did inquire about energy levels found that 87.5 percent of patients were fatigued.[16]

Methotrexate

Methotrexate interferes with the work of folic acid (also called folate) — a B vitamin needed to replicate cells. Like cyclophosphamide, methotrexate affects normal cells as well as cancer cells. If a high dose is used, oncologists sometimes need to follow it with leucovorin, a special form of folic acid. In theory, the leucovorin can stop the action of the methotrexate before it becomes too toxic.

Like cyclophosphamide, methotrexate can cause birth defects, menstrual dysfunction, and infertility. It also rules out breastfeeding. Sometimes it damages the liver, the lungs, and/or the kidneys.

The most common side effects from this drug (occurring in about one patient in ten) include oral ulcerations,* nausea, vomiting, and abdominal distress. The damage caused to the gastrointestinal tract suggests that methotrexate should not be taken by women with a past history of serious gastrointestinal diseases, such as ulcerative colitis, Crohn's disease, or ulcers.

---

*Oral ulcerations have been reported to heal quickly by simply rubbing 400 units of vitamin E on them twice per day, according to the May 1992 issue of *The American Journal of Medicine.*

Patients taking methotrexate often become tired and may experience malaise, headaches, and diarrhea. As with cyclophosphamide, WBC production can be seriously impaired, leading to an increased risk of infection. It may be dangerous to take this drug if an active infection already exists.

Patients receiving methotrexate should consult their oncologists about possible drug interaction problems. Of primary concern are nonsteroidal anti-inflammatory drugs like aspirin or Tylenol. The interaction may be dangerous. Self-administered folic acid supplements are also of concern, because they might interfere with the action of the drug. It's unclear whether the small amount of folic acid (usually 400 micrograms) found in multivitamins is enough to be problematic. Discuss it with your oncologist.

Fluorouracil

Fluorouracil has the rather ominously ironic trade name "5-FU." Like cyclophosphamide and methotrexate, it blocks cellular replication. And like the others, it does not selectively target cancer cells but affects everything.

Drug reference books consider fluorouracil a highly toxic drug with a narrow margin of safety. They warn that the drug should be discontinued when any of the following side effects occurs: inflammation of the mouth, a large drop in the WBC count, intractable vomiting, diarrhea, gastrointestinal ulceration and bleeding, or hemorrhage from any site. Yet, some of these problems (like inflammation of the mouth, diarrhea, and a drop in the WBC count) are relatively common and are also associated with the companion drugs given with fluorouracil. Other common side effects are inflammation of the esophagus, loss of appetite, and nausea.

Substantial numbers of patients on fluorouracil experience hair loss and dermatitis. The drug is also suspected of causing birth defects. As with the other drugs, breastfeeding should be ruled out.

General Considerations About Toxicity

We have looked at the action and toxicity of each of the three drugs when taken separately. Much is also known about their toxicity when used together. An English study reported the percentage of patients experiencing the following side effects when on CMF:[17]

- Nausea/vomiting (82 percent)
- Hair loss (65 percent)
- A large drop in white blood cells (62 percent)
- Anxiety or depression (over 50 percent)
- Inflammation of the mouth (32 percent)
- Inflammation of the lining of the eyelids (31 percent)
- Diarrhea (22 percent)
- A dangerous drop in white blood cells (8 percent)
- Inflammation of the bladder (6 percent)

The Ludwig group of breast cancer researchers has reported that deaths and life-threatening infections occur in fewer than 1 percent of patients taking CMF.[18] This prominent research group has reported that, overall, CMF led to "mild to moderate" toxicity in 78 percent and "severe" toxicity in 8.5 percent of patients taking these drugs.[19] However, the Interstudy Group, another leading assembly of researchers, reports severe or life-threatening toxicity (as measured by a drop in WBC counts) in every third patient.[20] These variations may be due to differences in CMF dosages. The trend has been toward *increasing* doses, which would increase toxicity.

Even the studies that do list toxicities generally don't talk about weight gain, sexual dysfunction, insomnia, and anxiety — all of which occur. They also frequently don't address permanent infertility.

Weight gain occurs in most women taking chemotherapy for breast cancer. One study that did investigate this side effect found it in 69 percent of women.[21] Average amounts of weight gained vary from study to study, but are typically in the nine- to thirteen-pound range. Dr. John Camoriano from the Scottsdale, Arizona, Mayo Clinic found that almost 20 percent of premenopausal women taking chemotherapy gained an average of 22 pounds.[22] The reasons for this weight gain remain unclear, though it occurs more in premenopausal women.[23]

Sexual problems can also result from chemotherapy. Though they are apparently common, they're generally ignored in the toxicity sections of the major chemotherapy trials. Helen Kaplan from the Human Sexuality Program at Cornell University Medical Center says the following, in a letter to the *Lancet:*

> We are seeing more and more women (and couples) complaining of the sexual side-effects of these treatments. Chemotherapy can have devastating effects on female sexual response (desire, vaginal lubrication, and orgasm) because most chemotherapy used in the United States for the adjuvant treatment of early breast cancer interferes with the production of oestrogen and testosterone. A deficiency of oestrogen, which is desirable for patients with oestrogen-sensitive tumours, produces a chemical menopause with atrophic changes in the vagina [which can cause pain with intercourse]. Chemotherapy can also interfere with female androgen [sex hormone] production, and we have found androgen-deficiency-related sexual complaints in a substantial number of patients. This androgen deficiency is marked by a loss of libido and a greatly diminished capacity for orgasm, changes that can be more devastating to women and their partners than the vaginal dryness produced by the lack of oestrogen or the loss of a breast. Unfortunately many women with the syndrome are misdiagnosed and are referred for psychosexual therapy, to which they are not amenable. . . . [T]his impairment of sex-hormone production can be permanent. . . .[24]

Rose Kushner says, "When oncologists give women their favorite combination of [chemotherapy], they are literally making healthy people sick, even though most evidence today indicates that the toxic regimens are of only marginal benefit to the vast majority of women who develop breast cancer — those who are postmenopausal."[25]

Having read this far, you may be tempted to give up the idea of chemotherapy altogether. Don't — at least not yet. It's true that some groups of women may be better off forgoing chemo. But for other subsets of patients, the benefits may outweigh the risks. Ultimately, the decision should be yours. You need to understand what possible benefits exist for you, given your specific situation, before saying "no" to drugs. The rest of this chapter provides an explanation of what is known about who is apt to benefit and who is not. We'll also consider how likely these potential benefits are.

CHEMOTHERAPY AND NODE-NEGATIVE WOMEN

By definition, stage I patients have no cancer in their lymph nodes — they are node-negative. It is possible to be node-negative yet be at a higher stage if the breast tumor was greater than 2 centimeters (0.8 inch). Most of the research looking at node-negative women does not divide patients into stage I and stage II. If you are node-negative, this section applies to you even if your cancer has technically been called stage II disease.

Node-negative patients with very small tumors — less than 1 centimeter (0.4 inch) — stand an 86 percent chance of being cured simply by surgery or the combination of surgery and radiation, according to most research (see "A Review of the Node-Negative Trials" later in this chapter). But, if all node-negative patients are considered together, the cure rate from surgery or the combination of surgery and radiation alone is only about 70 percent. Thus, three node-negative patients in ten will eventually suffer a recurrence. An average of less than one of these three will be helped by chemotherapy.

In 1992, the *Lancet* published an enormous compilation of studies put together by the Early Breast Cancer Trialists' Collaborative Group. In this, the largest report ever published, most node-negative patients lived, with or without chemotherapy; and, of course, some died either way. But only one out of every twenty-five node-negative patients taking chemotherapy was alive at ten years as a result of the chemotherapy when compared with similar patients not taking chemo.[26]

Earlier in this chapter we discussed extended disease-free survival without any increase in life expectancy. A 1991 review reports this pattern specifically for node-negative patients taking chemotherapy.[27]

We might conclude that chemotherapy is a poor choice for node-negative women. But let's take a closer look: In the same way that stage I patients with very small tumors have a much better than 70 percent chance of cure, it follows that other node-negative women must have a significantly worse than 70 percent chance. Oncologists are hoping to reserve chemotherapy for "high-risk" node-negative patients and avoid it in "low-risk" patients. The problem is deciding who falls into which group. Although we know that 90 percent of very low risk patients can be identified simply by tumor size, identifying high-risk patients is more complicated.

One factor found to increase the risk of a recurrence is ER-negative status (see Chapter 9). An early Italian study of ER-negative, node-negative patients found that chemotherapy doubled the chance of remaining disease-free.[28] The medical community was excited. But something was wrong: The group that did not receive chemo fared much worse than similar patients in similar studies.[29,30] In other words, what made the Italian results dramatic was not how well the patients did on chemo, but how poorly they did without it. The results of this study have therefore been viewed with skepticism.

A Review of the Node-Negative Trials

Late in February 1989, a week before Cathy was diagnosed, the *New England Journal of Medicine* published the results of a series of trials using chemotherapy for node-negative women. The studies led to a dramatic increase in the use of chemotherapy for node-negative patients. In 1992 those trials were partially superseded by the giant Early Breast Cancer Trialists' Collaborative Group report that appeared in the *Lancet*.[31] Before looking at the *Lancet* report, let's go over the *New England Journal* studies that led to the increased use of chemo for node-negative women.

In one of the *New England Journal* studies, the Ludwig Trial V, one woman in every twenty-five was spared a recurrence in the first forty-two months as a result of CMF.[32] The other twenty-four still paid the physical, emotional, and financial costs of chemotherapy without any benefit. There was no survival advantage from taking chemo. These dismal results were considered a success by mainstream medicine.

The same issue of the *New England Journal* reported Protocol B-13 of the National Surgical Adjuvant Breast and Bowel Project (NSABP).[33] The patients in this trial were ER- and node-negative.* After five years, one woman in eleven was spared a recurrence as a result of taking chemo.[34] But even after seven years, there was still no overall survival advantage.[35]

The authors say the benefit of increased disease-free survival was achieved "with a highly acceptable level of toxicity."[36] Nausea and vomiting were the only very common side effects because cyclophosphamide, the most toxic drug usually used, was excluded. But all the usual toxicities did occur to some women. To whom are these side effects highly acceptable?

The NSABP researchers claimed that the prognosis of all node-negative patients is poor enough to justify chemotherapy,[37] but most scientists disagree. A review of the research finds that 86 percent of stage I patients with very small tumors (1 centimeter or less) remain disease-free even without chemo for at least twenty years.[38]

Another large trial, the Intergroup Study, appeared in the same issue of the *New England Journal,* looking at high-risk** node-negative patients.[39] The best results were reported in this trial. Those who were followed five years had a disease-free survival rate of 83 percent in the chemo group versus 61 percent without chemo. Thus, one woman in four or five was spared a recurrence.[40] But these results were balanced by the fact that severe or even life-threatening toxicity occurred in every third woman.[41]

---

*These women were first given methotrexate and later fluorouracil. Cyclophosphamide, the most toxic of the CMF combination, was left out.

**They defined "high-risk" as either being ER-negative or having a large (at least 3 centimeters) breast tumor.

As a result of these *New England Journal* articles, oncologists in the United States began to use more chemotherapy for treating node-negative women. The National Cancer Institute issued a clinical alert advising the use of chemo for node-negative women. Bernard Fisher of the NSABP said, "there should be no vacillation whatsoever. Every patient should either go into a clinical trial or should be given the therapies."[42] In a sense, this means it's acceptable for a doctor to withhold chemotherapy if the patient is being used as a guinea pig in a research trial, but otherwise it's unethical. I find this a troubling philosophical position.

Many breast cancer researchers from other countries have felt differently about chemo for node-negative women. English researchers from Guy's Hospital in London say, "there can be no justification for [chemotherapy's] widespread introduction in all patients with node-negative breast cancer."[43]

A group of Canadian scientists concluded that benefits "have been modest and may not outweigh the cost and toxic effects of such therapy. Routine use does not seem to be justified."[44] After looking at the results of many studies, these Canadian doctors found that node-negative women generally fare much better than those studied in the *New England Journal*. Therefore, the *New England Journal* reports used to justify the claim that virtually all node-negative women should receive chemo may really pertain to just high-risk node-negative women.

Even some Americans have had doubts about using chemo indiscriminately in node-negative women. Edward Mansour, the principal investigator of the Intergroup Study, advises patients to avoid chemotherapy "if they're going to live free of disease anyway, which most node-negative patients will do."[45] K. C. Lee, a Georgetown University doctor, says, "we will be forever subjecting the 70 percent of patients already cured by surgery or irradiation to the morbidity, mortality, and expense associated with treatment that they do not need. . . . I do not know how one can expect to give unnecessary treatment to 50,000 women each year in the United States."[46] Ten medical doctors from the Mayo Clinic said, "Clear-cut benefits for systemic therapy in [node-negative, small-tumor] breast cancers are not apparent in any of these trials."[47] Thomas Nealon Jr., from New York University, has said, "Good risk tumors of the breast do not require adjuvant therapy."[48] He followed a group of stage I patients with pathology reports suggesting low risk (see Chapter 3). Of his sixty patients, fifty-eight remained disease-free, including every woman who did not take chemotherapy. "Low risk node-negative tumors of the breast do not require adjuvant therapy. Recurrence is so rare, use of adjuvant therapy is not justified. In the few instances of recurrence the adjuvant therapy did not help."

Thus far, we might conclude the following: Chemotherapy helps some node-negative women; but if your chance of a recurrence is relatively small, it may not be worth the potential side effects or the risks. Such an approach seems reasonable, yet information about which factors determine high or low risk in node-negative patients has not been consistent.[49] The problem is that everyone defines risk levels differently.

In 1992, at an international symposium of breast cancer researchers held in Switzerland, a node-negative woman at low risk was defined as having any of the following characteristics:[50]

- Noninvasive cancer (also called carcinoma *in situ*)
- A tumor 1 centimeter or less in size
- A cancer designated by the pathologist as tubular, colloid, mucinous, or papillary (see Chapter 3)

This international meeting concluded that women with any of these characteristics had too low a risk of recurrence to use chemotherapy. The same conference concluded that patients with tumors between 1 and 2 centimeters who were ER-positive and had a good grade (see Chapter 3) should take tamoxifen and not risk the side effects of chemotherapy.

In a presentation made to the American Society of Clinical Oncologists, researchers from Roswell Park Memorial Institute in Buffalo, New York, reported that their patients with tumors less than 1 centimeter had an excellent prognosis without chemo (96 percent survival at seven years and 91 percent disease-free survival at seven years). "These data suggest that [such patients] are highly curable by [surgery] alone, and the authors believe that these women are not appropriate candidates for adjuvant therapy until such time as subgroups at high risk of recurrence can be identified."[51] The same researchers have reported elsewhere that some other node-negative women also don't need chemotherapy.[52] They studied women with tumors between 1.1 and 2 centimeters considered "well" or "moderately differentiated" by the pathologist (see Chapter 3). In their study, well over 90 percent of these patients were disease-free after seven years without chemo. Again, this suggests that the risks of chemo are not justified for these women.

In contrast, Gianni Bonadonna, the principal investigator in the Italian trials, strongly advocates using chemotherapy for many node-negative patients. However, even he draws the line at women with tumors less than two centimeters who are also ER-positive and/or grade 1 (see Chapter 3). He writes, "The vast majority of these women can be spared chemotherapy."[53]

The hunt for other groups of node-negative patients who might consider avoiding chemo has caused researchers at the University of Virginia Health Sciences Center in Charlottesville to look at the patient's age.[54] After a seven-year follow-up, these researchers report that node-negative women older than 70 are considerably more likely to die of other causes than of the breast cancer. Such a finding makes the recommendation to use chemotherapy in anyone over 70 a questionable idea at best.

Even the editorial accompanying the 1989 *New England Journal* articles said, "it must be concluded that relatively few patients (4 to 15 percent) benefited, at least in terms of remaining free of detectable disease."[55] The editorial warned against the widespread use of chemotherapy in node-negative patients, arguing "that the cost considerably outweighs the benefits of treating all node negative patients, especially in the absence of a proved survival benefit." So ironically, at the same time conventional medicine in America was being swayed by the articles published by the *New England Journal,* the *New England Journal* itself was advising caution.

Three years after the *New England Journal* reports, the *Lancet* published a much larger collaborative study.[56] It included all the February 1989 *New England Journal* reports plus many others. The results of this effort found that 61.5 percent of node-negative women taking chemotherapy were free of all breast cancer versus 54.5 percent without chemo after more than 10 years. (These poor disease-free survival percentages suggest, as with the *New England Journal* reports, that women in this collaborative study were at higher-than-average risk.) Survival rates during this same period of time were 67.2 percent for women taking chemo and 63.2 percent for women not given chemo. This means for every 25 women given chemotherapy, only one life was spared. Despite these modest gains, the 1992 *Lancet* report was considered yet more evidence that node-negative women should take chemotherapy.

Thus far, the talk about apparent benefits of chemo in node-negative patients has not considered quality of life. Most researchers don't factor in this very important issue when comparing chemo results to a control group not receiving chemo.

What happens when researchers do bother to figure in side effects? An independent analysis of the 1992 *Lancet* data considered quality of life.[57] This analysis found that node-negative women aged 75 had an average gain in quality-adjusted life of only 1.8 months at a cost of more than $44,000 per person. When months of active life were compared, the benefit decreased to only two weeks at a cost of more than $86,000! Why are the gains so small? The main reason is simple: Few women avoid a recurrence as a result of the chemo, but virtually all suffer side effects. When the suffering of the many is subtracted from the benefit of the few, the average benefit is remarkably meager. We can see how statistics about overall survival or disease-free survival can be misleading when they don't consider quality of life.

A few other scientists have realized the need to factor in quality-adjusted time. A reexamination of patients from the Ludwig V trial considered this issue.[58] When quality of life was ignored, chemo appeared effective. But when quality-adjusted time was studied, life expectancy increased only 1.5 months for postmenopausal and 2.8 months for premenopausal women as a result of chemo.

One of the justifications for using chemo in node-negative women has been the assumption that the moderate increases in disease-free survival shown in many studies will inevitably lead to increases in overall survival. However, this hasn't usually happened. As noted earlier in this chapter, there are reasons to suspect it won't happen. Ian Tannock, of Princess Margaret Hospital in Toronto, has shown that trials done with node-positive women are frequently not nearly so impressive at 10 years as they are at earlier points in time. The same might ultimately prove true for node-negative women. Tannock questions the assumption of many researchers that a long-term increase in survival in the node-negative chemo groups is all but inevitable.[59]

The cost of treating women who will not benefit from chemotherapy has been estimated as $500,000,000 per year for the United States alone.[60] The personal cost to these women is more important, though often unmentioned. Is it worth it? Once in possession of the available information, you have a right to be included in the decision.

Summary of Chemotherapy Results with Node-Negative Women

- Most (almost 70 percent) node-negative patients are cured without chemo.
- Most node-negative patients who would ultimately die from breast cancer will not be cured by chemotherapy.
- Chemo modestly increases the disease-free survival for node-negative patients.
- Chemo increases overall survival very modestly for node-negative patients.
- Gains in disease-free survival are much less impressive when toxicity from the chemo is considered. Most studies reporting good results do not factor in toxicity.
- Some node-negative patients are at such low risk of recurrence

that most researchers do not feel chemo is justified. Typically these women have at least one of the following:

- Tumors 1 centimeter or smaller
- Tumors between 1 and 2 centimeters with good indicators such as ER-positive status and good grade
- Tumors described by the pathologist as tubular, colloid, mucinous, or papillary (forms of breast cancer unlikely to be fatal)

If you are node-negative and do not fall into one of these groups, you may be at higher than normal risk of a recurrence. Even so, you might not benefit from chemo after surgery and/or radiation. Unfortunately we don't have a crystal ball. Chemo might help you. There is no simple answer to the question of whether to use or avoid chemotherapy for higher-risk node-negative patients, though many medical doctors in the United States are leaning toward using it. No one can say ahead of time whether you are the woman who will benefit or even to what extent you will suffer the side effects. With either choice you gamble.

Cathy ultimately opted to do neither tamoxifen nor chemotherapy. Because we lack information about both nodal and ER status, it has been impossible to accurately assess her risk of recurrence. Perhaps we've been lucky. But when I think of all the problems we avoided by her decision, I feel that women have a right to "just say no." The assessment of your risk should be discussed with your oncologist before you make the decision to undergo or avoid chemotherapy.

An Alternative to Chemotherapy

Let us assume that you are node-negative but not in a particularly low risk group and are therefore seriously considering chemotherapy. If you are in your 40s and are premenopausal, you may have an important, less invasive alternative to chemotherapy: surgical removal of the ovaries. This option is not frequently taken; but, according to the massive collaborative

Lancet study, it is just as effective.[61,62] It may actually be even more effective for some women and it has fewer side effects than chemotherapy. If you are interested in considering this option, jump to "Ovarian Ablation" on page 84.

CHEMOTHERAPY, OVARIAN ABLATION, AND NODE-POSITIVE WOMEN

As stated in preceding chapters, this book is limited to discussing early-stage breast cancer. Generally, this means stage I and II disease. Stage I means no nodal involvement and a breast tumor of 2 centimeters or less. Stage II includes some node-negative women who have tumors larger than 2 centimeters and women with "limited nodal involvement." "Limited" means that all cancerous lymph nodes are movable and limited to the ipsilateral (same side) axilla (armpit). This section will discuss the use of chemotherapy to treat women with limited nodal involvement, which, for the sake of simplicity, we'll call "node-positive" disease.

When groups of node-positive patients are followed for many years, the percentage cured by surgery and/or radiation alone is sometimes under 50 percent. Because these odds are far from ideal, if you are node-positive you may need to consider taking higher risks (like the side effects of chemotherapy) in your hunt for a cure. Fortunately, chemotherapy is usually more effective in node-positive women.

Chemotherapy is particularly effective in node-positive, premenopausal women. There is evidence that premenopausal women have more rapidly growing cancers.[63] If cancer cells are replicating faster than healthy cells, the chemo can destroy the cancer before it does too much damage to the rest of the body. Most conventional researchers and medical doctors agree that women who are node-positive and premenopausal should take chemotherapy. This section will review the benefits of chemotherapy for node-positive, premenopausal women. We will also consider a conventional alternative to chemotherapy that appears more successful than chemo in some women.

In addition, we'll evaluate the effects of chemo if you're node-positive and postmenopausal, a group that benefits a little from taking chemotherapy. If you are both node-positive and postmenopausal, the main question is, Can you forgo the use of chemo in favor of the less toxic tamoxifen, or does it make sense to consider both treatments?

A Review of the Node-Positive Trials

The largest compilation of node-positive chemo studies appeared as part of the *Lancet* collaborative trial.[64] At five years, 53.5 percent of the node-positive women taking chemo were still disease-free versus 44.2 percent not taking chemo. ("disease-free survival" counts only women who have no recurrence of breast cancer while "overall survival" counts all women who remain alive, even if the cancer has returned.) After ten years these disease-free numbers fell to 38.5 percent with chemo and 29.8 percent without it.* Thus, one woman out of every eleven or twelve taking chemo was spared a recurrence. If we look at overall survival statistics, at five years the numbers were about the same with or without chemo (66.5 percent versus 63.3 percent); but beyond ten years, significantly more women were alive who took chemo (46.6 percent) versus those who did not (39.8 percent). This translates into one woman in fifteen remaining alive at more than ten years as a result of chemotherapy.

When this collaborative report is divided by age or menopausal status, it's clear that premenopausal women benefited much more from chemo than did postmenopausal women. (Although the figures for pre- and postmenopausal women include all patients regardless of their nodal status, most of the women in these trials were node-positive.)

---

*The way "early breast cancer" is defined by these researchers, stage III patients with advanced nodal involvement or very large (greater than 5 cm) tumors are not excluded; therefore, if you have stage II disease, your chances of survival and disease-free survival are better than these numbers indicate.

If we look at all premenopausal women regardless of how long they were followed, 67 percent survived taking chemotherapy versus 60 percent not taking it. Chemo saved a life for every fourteen women. Disease-free survival was 57.2 percent among those taking chemo versus 47.8 percent among those not taking chemo. Thus almost one premenopausal woman in ten was spared a recurrence as a result of chemo.

For postmenopausal women chemo was much less useful in reducing the death rate: 71.5 percent survived with CMF versus 69 percent without it. In terms of disease-free survival, the numbers were 63 percent with chemo versus 56.5 percent without it. For postmenopausal women in their 50s, one life was saved for every fifty women taking chemo. For women in their 60s, a life was saved for every thirty-four women taking these drugs. These numbers strongly suggest to me that postmenopausal women should consider tamoxifen rather than agree to chemotherapy.

Ovarian Ablation

One of the trials in the compiled *Lancet* data was the Manchester/Guy's Hospital study.[65] Initial publication of this report revealed a controversial finding. The positive effect of chemotherapy at Guy's Hospital happened in premenopausal women only. On closer inspection, most of this effect happened in premenopausal women in their forties who permanently lost their menstrual cycle as a result of taking chemotherapy. When this group is viewed separately, the results are dramatic. The five-year survival rates were 74.5 percent taking chemo versus 37 percent without chemo. Women in their 40s who were already postmenopausal before they took the chemo were not helped by chemotherapy. A previous Italian trial found the same pattern. Others have also acknowledged that premenopausal women who become amenorrheic do better with chemo than do premenopausal women who retain their menstrual cycle.[66]

Does chemotherapy help premenopausal women simply by destroying their ovaries and thus making them postmenopausal? The Guy's Hospital researchers say their results "strongly suggest that menstrual status rather than an arbitrary cutoff age should be used both in analyses and in selecting those patients who should receive adjuvant chemotherapy." Most major American trials can't address this concern because patients are divided into groups on the basis of their 50th birthday — not their menopausal status.

Why should premenopausal women from the Guy's Hospital study who permanently lost their period as a result of chemo do so well? Cessation of the menstrual cycle means dramatically reducing the production of estrogen. Estrogen is known to feed the cancer. The fact that most studies find chemo more effective in premenopausal women suggests that at least part of the effectiveness of these drugs results from the destruction of the ovaries' ability to make estrogen. (Ovaries in postmenopausal women no longer make significant amounts of estrogen.)

The removal of ovaries or the loss of ovarian function as a result of anything other than normal menopause is called oophorectomy, ovarian ablation, or castration. When chemotherapy is responsible, the effect is called "chemical castration." (This term is found in the medical journals, though your oncologist is not likely to use it to your face.) If you are premenopausal, you might find the idea of such a procedure shocking. But if the primary therapeutic effect of chemo comes from destroying ovarian function, it may make sense to consider removal of the ovaries before agreeing to chemotherapy.

Keep in mind, for women over 40, the chemo will also typically destroy ovarian function. For women younger than 40, chemotherapy frequently does not permanently eliminate the menstrual cycle. But for both groups, surgically removing the ovaries rather than taking chemotherapy will spare nausea, vomiting, loss of immune function, hair loss, increased risk of other cancers, etc. To say this another way, if chemical castration is primarily what's helping premenopausal women over age 40 who take chemo, ovarian ablation should at least be considered as an alternative.

The 1992 *Lancet* compilation of many trials followed several thousand women who were assigned either to a control group or to a group receiving surgical or radiation-induced ovarian ablation.[67]

For women under 50, ovarian ablation was just as effective as chemotherapy. Significant reductions in mortality were reported; these held up and even improved after the first nine years.

A *Lancet* editorial acknowledged that ovarian ablation worked as well as chemotherapy for premenopausal women.[68] It went on to say that this finding provides further evidence for the notion that chemotherapy in premenopausal women acts largely via chemical castration.

Disease-free survival in node-positive women below age 50 (meaning mostly premenopausal women) was about 50 percent with ovarian ablation versus 37 percent without it, after ten years. Overall survival figures at more than 15 years were 49.6 percent with ovarian ablation versus 36.5 percent without it.

Recently the Guy's Hospital report, in combination with a Scottish trial, has been updated and published in the *Lancet*.[69] Once again, it was shown that, overall, for premenopausal women, ovarian ablation (from radiation or surgery) was as useful as chemotherapy. However, this new report goes a step further.

These researchers looked at estrogen receptor levels and discovered a clear pattern: The higher the ER level, the better ovarian ablation did compared with chemotherapy. (See Chapters 3 and 9 for discussion of estrogen receptors.) For women with ER levels from 0 to 4, chemotherapy was significantly better than ovarian ablation. For women with levels between 5 and 19, this pattern still existed, though the difference was somewhat smaller. For women with ER levels between 20 and 99, ovarian ablation actually appeared to be more effective than chemotherapy, though again the difference did not reach statistical significance. But for women with ER levels at or above 100, ovarian ablation was dramatically more effective than chemotherapy (the chance of a recurrence dropped by more than half); though once again, due to small numbers of women in this group, the difference did not reach statistical significance.

The issue of how estrogen receptor levels affect the efficacy of chemo versus ovarian ablation may be interesting, but normally scientists don't put much emphasis on the results of one trial. However, because the Guy's Hospital/Scottish Trial confirms the conclusions about ovarian ablation found in the 1992 *Lancet* report, which combined data from many trials, and because the new report showed that the efficacy of ovarian ablation compared to chemo was directly proportional to ER levels, it seems doubtful that the results constitute pure chance. Frankly, until more is known, I think the results of this report should be taken very seriously.

To summarize, it appears that premenopausal women benefit more from ovarian ablation than from chemotherapy if their ER levels are high. The higher the level, the better the surgery worked compared to chemotherapy. Levels at or above 20 are considered the beginning of "high" by the definition of these researchers. Conversely, it now appears that women who are ER-negative or mildly positive (between 0 and 19) are helped more by chemotherapy than by ovarian ablation. For these women, according to the new trial, ovarian ablation might be less effective despite the "overall" results being equivalent between chemo and ovarian ablation.

Of course, like every other issue involving chemotherapy choices, this story has two sides. A few studies report that at least some of the women helped by chemo are postmenopausal;[70] therefore, it's clear that the therapeutic effect for these women is not a function of chemical castration. But this begs the question: How much of chemotherapy's effect in premenopausal women is due to ovarian destruction? The answer appears to be "most," according to the *Lancet* overview.

Of course, destroying the ovaries or removing them also creates problems — including increased risks of cardiovascular disease and osteoporosis, as well as vaginal dryness and severe hot flashes. Risks of cardiovascular disease and osteoporosis can be reduced by lifestyle modifications, most of which you will already be making if you follow the prevention guidelines in Chapters 12–14. And remember, these same risks exist when cessation in ovarian function results from chemotherapy. In other words, the chemo can do the same thing and for the same reason — either way, ovaries stop functioning. The *Lancet* concluded, "Ovarian ablation should be seriously considered as an alternative to adjuvant chemotherapy in premenopausal women."[71]

Combined Therapies: Chemo and Tamoxifen

Recently, NSABP researchers and others have suggested small gains when chemotherapy is combined with tamoxifen in the same patient.* Although the *Lancet* collaborative report also suggests that the two therapies might be useful in combination, other trials don't support this idea. In fact, one review of the chemo-plus-tamoxifen trials found that, for every study with good results, there was another reporting the combination to be no better than tamoxifen alone.[72]

As an example of this confusion, let's look at an Italian trial that studied node-positive, ER-positive patients given chemo, tamoxifen, or both.[73] This study claimed that the combination of both therapies was better than either alone. Yet, overall survival results were virtually the same for tamoxifen versus tamoxifen plus chemotherapy. In fact, more women with three or fewer positive nodes survived with tamoxifen alone than with tamoxifen plus chemotherapy.

Because of the extensive toxicity, adding chemotherapy to a regimen of tamoxifen should be done only if it produces clear and obvious advantages — not just minor but statistically significant improvements. And most of the trials that claim an "advantage" for using the combination do not factor in quality of life. I'm concerned that marginal improvements resulting from the combination would disappear if quality of life were considered.

The positive talk about combining therapies (from the NSABP and others) is beginning to affect the thinking of some oncologists. If you're considering taking both drug regimens, read

---

*Chapter 9 includes a more extensive discussion about using both therapies to treat the same patient. We examine the combination of chemo and tamoxifen in this (node-positive) section because very few node-negative patients are offered both therapies.

Chapter 9, focusing on the section called "Tamoxifen and Chemotherapy." Keep in mind that taking this combination will expose you to both sets of side effects. At least for now, the benefits of such an approach seem relatively speculative.

CHEMOTHERAPY FOR WOMEN OVER 70

Although postmenopausal women have been studied in many trials, most of these patients were between 50 and 69. Much less is known regarding the use of chemotherapy in older women. The huge *Lancet* collaborative study included so few women over 70 that the authors say conclusions should not be drawn for this age group.[74] However, chemotherapy did not help the few older women studied in the *Lancet* report. Moreover, it obviously becomes more difficult to withstand the side effects of chemotherapy as you grow older. Fortunately, tamoxifen seems to help older women even when they are ER-negative (see Chapter 9). In most cases, therefore, it seems appropriate for early-stage breast cancer patients over the age of 70 to take tamoxifen and forgo chemotherapy, at least until more is known.

CHEMOTHERAPY TO AVOID MASTECTOMY IN PATIENTS WITH LARGE TUMORS

Recently, researchers have been considering using chemotherapy before surgery as a way to shrink large tumors (3 centimeters or more). They hope that mastectomy can be avoided and a simple lumpectomy can follow the chemo.

The Italian researcher Gianni Bonadonna has reported that preoperative CMF can successfully shrink large tumors to the point where lumpectomy becomes a viable option.[75] He reports that 91 percent of large tumors (initially less than 5 centimeters) were sufficiently reduced in size to allow for lumpectomy.[76] In fact, in 8 of 220 women, the tumor simply disappeared.

The obvious questions are what preoperative chemotherapy does to survival and disease-free survival numbers and how it compares with the more common use of chemo several weeks after surgery. Unfortunately, too little preoperative chemotherapy has been done to answer these questions yet. As a result, preoperative chemo may allow for more limited surgery but must still be considered experimental.

AN OVERVIEW

The news media and your oncologist may be very upbeat about chemotherapy. In fact, this chapter may well be the only information about chemo you'll get that does not sound like an advertisement for these drugs.

How can chemo be championed as a great step forward when the overall results appear so modest? Indraneel Mittra, a Bombay surgeon, has considered this issue in the prestigious *British Medical Journal*.[77] He comes to the conclusion that researchers whose studies show little or no benefit convert their data to a "positive" outcome by hunting through the numbers after the studies are completed to see if there is any way to divide women so that some group is created that appears to have benefited. Researchers officially call this "retrospective subset analysis," but it is unofficially considered "massaging the data" to make them say what you want them to.

Mittra goes on to show that by hunting through various trials, it is also possible to "create" groups of women who did much worse by taking chemotherapy than those who didn't. Although these results are as meaningful as those touted in the press and by oncologists, they receive little or no attention. This thoughtful article concludes by saying we shouldn't simply focus on identifying high-risk patients and assume that they should all take chemo. Rather, we need to concentrate on who is being helped by chemo. The two groups are not necessarily the same. In other words, why take chemotherapy just because you are at high risk if it appears that the chemo wouldn't help you?

As we have acknowledged, virtually every group of early-stage women obtains at least some on-paper benefit from taking chemo when side effects are not considered. If you are both node-positive and premenopausal, the benefits of chemotherapy may outweigh the risks, though the option of ovarian ablation needs to be considered very carefully as an alternative. If you do not fit into this group, you might well decide the risks outweigh the benefits. Regardless of which group you're in, it may be useful to reread this chapter, jot down your specific questions, and discuss them with your oncologist before making a decision.

The following is a review of who is helped most by chemotherapy:

- Premenopausal women more than postmenopausal women
- Premenopausal women who permanently lose ovarian function more than those who retain a menstrual cycle
- Node-positive women more than node-negative women
- Women who had tumors with a poor grade more than women whose tumors were given a good grade

Most of the benefits from chemotherapy occur within the first three or four years from the time of diagnosis. It's true that small improvements in overall survival sometimes show up well past this point. But beyond the fourth year, disease-free differences between groups receiving and not receiving chemo don't usually grow any larger. Therefore, if you refrain from using chemotherapy and survive disease-free through the first four years, you've spared yourself the multiple problems associated with these drugs and probably would not have benefited had you made the opposite decision.

Cathy is now well beyond the fourth year. In the seemingly endless line of roulette wheels a breast cancer patient must spin, it's comforting for her to know that whatever else happens, she probably spun right when she declined chemotherapy.

Before leaving the topic of chemotherapy, I should acknowledge that it has not been possible to review here every report relevant to this chapter. Moreover, the research is in constant transition. By the time you read this, it's possible a new study applicable to women in your situation will just have been published. For these reasons, make sure you carefully discuss the issues raised here with your doctors. Considering multiple points of view can be confusing, but it can also ultimately provide you with the most solid foundation from which to make your decision.

Making that decision depends not just on nodal, menopausal, and ER status. It also depends on your age, your overall health, what risks you feel are appropriate, and what potential benefits you consider large enough to take seriously.

Finally, I'd like to move away from the statistics in order to look at the broader picture. In the introductory remarks to "The Murders in the Rue Morgue," Edgar Allan Poe makes a distinction between mere calculation and the ability to analyze. He chides the Paris police for being able to go through multiple surface calculations without standing back from the data and seeing what's really going on. I believe this analogy can be used to describe chemo researchers studying breast cancer. Clearly, some women are helped. Nonetheless, if we look at the big picture, chemotherapy is a terrible treatment that, in centuries to come, may be viewed with as much horror as we view the use of mercurials or the practice of drilling holes in the head to let out evil spirits.

In *The Politics of Cancer,* Samuel Epstein reports that strong ties exist between the makers of chemotherapy drugs and the people in the hierarchies of the National Cancer Institute and the American Cancer Society who make decisions about how our research dollars are spent.[78] This relationship is unlikely to change in the near future. In fact, the recent call by women's groups to increase funding for breast cancer research may well simply lead to more studies splitting hairs over minor variations about which day to administer the drugs, how many months to do it for, whether this drug should precede that one, and so on. Rather than continuing to spend endless dollars chasing down these details, wouldn't it be more profitable to put our research dollars into other areas? The real question is, more profitable for whom? Continuing to prescribe and study therapies that lead to small but statistically significant gains is certainly not resulting in major payoffs for breast cancer patients.

Maybe, as individuals, we can't change the future course of breast cancer research. For the moment, you're stuck with your diagnosis and need to sort through the available information, much of it coming from those who are philosophically wedded to the belief that this dangerous therapy should be embraced readily and universally. Chemo does remain the right course for some women, despite its drawbacks. You may have a difficult decision in front of you. We wish you good luck.

References

1. Gelber, R. D., et al. Adjuvant treatment for breast cancer: the overview. *BMJ* 1992;304:859–60.

2. Kushner, R. Is aggressive adjuvant chemotherapy the Halsted radical of the '80s? *CA* 1984;34:345–51.

3. Smigel, K. Experts agree to disagree on adjuvant therapy for breast cancer. *J Natl Cancer Inst* 1990;82:640–1.

4. Henderson, I. C. Breast cancer therapy — the price of success. *N Engl J Med* 1992;326:1774–5 [editorial].

5. Mittra, I. Has adjuvant treatment of breast cancer had an unfair trial? *BMJ* 1990;301:1317–9.

6. Kushner, R. Is aggressive adjuvant chemotherapy the Halsted radical of the '80s? *CA* 1984;34:345–51.

7. Fisher, B., et al. A randomized clinical trial evaluating sequential methotrexate and fluorouracil in the treatment of patients with node-negative breast cancer who have estrogen-receptor-negative tumors. *N Engl J Med* 1989;3320:473–8.

8. Nealon, T. F., Jr. Low grade tumors of the breast do not require adjuvant therapy. American Cancer Society's Thirty-second Science Writers' Seminar, Daytona Beach, Florida, March 27, 1990.

9. Goldhirsch A., et al. Effect of systemic adjuvant treatment on first sites of breast cancer relapse. *Lancet* 1994;343:377–81.

10. Noguchi, S., et al. Influence of adjuvant chemotherapy for operable breast cancer on results of treatment at relapse. *Oncology* 1989;46:69–73.

11. Facelmann, K. A. Easing the sting of chemotherapy. *Sci News* 1989;135:238.

12. Redd, W. H., et al. Nausea induced by mental images of chemotherapy. *Cancer* 1993;72:629–36.

13. Curtis, R. E., et al. Risk of leukemia after chemotherapy and radiation treatment for breast cancer. *N Engl J Med* 1992;326:1745–51.

14. Andersson, M., et al. High risk of therapy-related leukemia and preleukemia after therapy with prednimustine, methotrexate, 5-fluorouracil, mitoxantrone, and tamoxifen for advanced breast cancer. *Cancer* 1990;65:2460–4.

15. Arriagada, R., and L. E. Rutqvist. Adjuvant chemotherapy in early breast cancer and incidence of new primary malignancies. *Lancet* 1991;338:535–8.

16. Tierney, A. J., et al. Side effects expected and experienced by women receiving chemotherapy for breast cancer. *BMJ* 1991;302:272–3.

17. Howell, A., et al. Controlled trial of adjuvant chemotherapy with cyclophosphamide, methotrexate, and fluorouracil for breast cancer. *Lancet* 1984;ii:307–11.

18. Ludwig Breast Cancer Study Group. Prolonged disease-free survival after one course of perioperative adjuvant chemotherapy for node-negative breast cancer. *N Engl J Med* 1989;320:491–6.

19. Ludwig Breast Cancer Study Group. Toxic effects of early adjuvant chemotherapy for breast cancer. *Lancet* 1983;ii:542–4.

20. Mansour, E. G., et al. Efficacy of adjuvant chemotherapy in high-risk node-negative breast cancer. *N Engl J Med* 1989;320:485–90.

21. Levine, E. G., et al. Weight gain with breast cancer adjuvant treatment. *Cancer* 1991;67:1954–9.

22. Smigel, K. Weight gain in breast cancer patients: a problem? *J Natl Cancer Inst* 1990;82:348–50.

23. Demark-Wahnefried, W., E. P. Winer, and B. K. Rimer. Why women gain weight with adjuvant chemotherapy for breast cancer. *J Clin Oncol* 1993;11:1418–29.

24. Kaplan, H. S. Adjuvant treatment in breast cancer. *Lancet* 1992;339:424 [letter].

25. Kushner, R. Is aggressive adjuvant chemotherapy the Halsted radical of the '80s? *CA* 1984;34:345–51.

26. Early Breast Cancer Trialists' Collaborative Group. Systemic treatment of early breast cancer by hormonal, cytotoxic, or immune therapy. *Lancet* 1992;339:1–15, 71–85.

27. Dorr, F. A., and M. A. Friedman. The role of chemotherapy in the management of primary breast cancer. *CA* 1991;41:231–41.

28. Bonadonna, G. Evolving concepts in the systemic adjuvant treatment of breast cancer. *Cancer Res* 1992;52:2127–37.

29. Fisher, B., et al. A randomized clinical trial evaluating sequential methotrexate and fluorouracil in the treatment of patients with node-negative breast cancer who have estrogen-receptor-negative tumors. *N Engl J Med* 1989;3320:473–8.

30. Mansour, E. G., et al. Efficacy of adjuvant chemotherapy in high-risk node-negative breast cancer. *N Engl J Med* 1989;320:485–90.

31. Early Breast Cancer Trialists' Collaborative Group. Systemic treatment of early breast cancer by hormonal, cytotoxic, or immune therapy. *Lancet* 1992;339:1–15, 71–85.

32. Ludwig Breast Cancer Study Group. Prolonged disease-free survival after one course of perioperative adjuvant chemotherapy for node-negative breast cancer. *N Engl J Med* 1989;320:491–6.

33. Fisher, B., et al. A randomized clinical trial evaluating sequential methotrexate and fluorouracil in the treatment of patients with node-negative breast cancer who have estrogen-receptor-negative tumors. *N Engl J Med* 1989;3320:473–8.

34. Fisher, B., et al. Recent developments in the use of systemic adjuvant therapy for the treatment of breast cancer. *Semin Oncol* 1992;19:263–77.

35. Glick, J. H., et al. Meeting highlights: adjuvant therapy for primary breast cancer. *J Natl Cancer Inst* 1992;84:1479–1485.

36. Fisher, B., et al. Recent developments in the use of systemic adjuvant therapy for the treatment of breast cancer. *Semin Oncol* 1992;19:263–77.

37. Fisher, B., et al. Systemic therapy in patients with node-negative breast cancer. *Ann Intern Med* 1989;111:703–12.

38. McGuire, W. L., and G. M. Clark. Prognostic factors and treatment decisions in axillary-node-negative breast cancer. *N Engl J Med* 1992;326:1756–61 [review].

39. Mansour, E. G., et al. Efficacy of adjuvant chemotherapy in high-risk node-negative breast cancer. *N Engl J Med* 1989;320:485–90.

40. Mansour, E. G., et al. Adjuvant therapy in node-negative breast cancer. Is it necessary for all patients? an Intergroup study. In *Adjuvant therapy of cancer,* ed. S. E. Salmon, Saunders, Philadelphia, 1990;VI:174–89.

41. Mansour, E. G., et al. Efficacy of adjuvant chemotherapy in high-risk node-negative breast cancer. *N Engl J Med* 1989;320:485–90.

42. Pollner, F. Data support adjuvant therapy. *Med World News* Mar 27, 1989; pp. 80, 85.

43. O'Reilly, S. M., and M. A. Richards. Node negative breast cancer — adjuvant chemotherapy should probably be reserved for patients at high risk of relapse. *BMJ* 1990;300:346–8 [review].

44. Ginsburg, A. D., et al. Systemic adjuvant therapy for node-negative breast cancer. *Can Med Assoc J* 1989;141:381–7 [review].

45. Pollner, F. Data support adjuvant therapy. *Med World News* Mar 27, 1989; pp. 80, 85.

46. Lee, K. C. Adjuvant therapy for node-negative breast cancer. *N Engl J Med* 1989;321:469 [letter].

47. Donohue, J. H., et al. Adjuvant therapy for node-negative breast cancer *N Engl J Med* 1989;321:470 [letter].

48. Nealon, T. F., Jr. Low grade tumors of the breast do not require adjuvant therapy. American Cancer Society's Thirty-second Science Writers' Seminar, Daytona Beach, Florida, March 27, 1990.

49. Ginsburg, A. D., et al. Systemic adjuvant therapy for node-negative breast cancer. *Can Med Assoc J* 1989;141:381–7 [review].

50. Glick, J. H., et al. Meeting highlights: adjuvant therapy for primary breast cancer. *J Natl Cancer Inst* 1992;84:1479–1485.

51. Rosner, D., and W. W. Lane. Node-negative minimal invasive breast cancer patients are not candidates for routine systemic adjuvant therapy. *Cancer* 1990;66:199–205.

52. Rosner, D., and W. W. Lane. Should all patients with node-negative breast cancer receive adjuvant therapy? *Cancer* 1991;68:1482–94.

53. Bonadonna, G. Evolving concepts in the systemic adjuvant treatment of breast cancer. *Cancer Res* 1992;52:2127–37.

54. Spaulding, C. A., et al. Node-negative breast carcinoma treated without adjuvant systemic therapy. *S Med J* 1992;85:355–64.

55. McGuire, W. L. Adjuvant therapy on node-negative breast cancer. *N Engl J Med* 1989;320:525–7 [editorial].

56. Early Breast Cancer Trialists' Collaborative Group. Systemic treatment of early breast cancer by hormonal, cytotoxic, or immune therapy. *Lancet* 1992;339:1–15, 71–85.

57. Desch, C. E., et al. Should the elderly receive chemotherapy for node-negative breast cancer? A cost-effectiveness analysis examining total active life-expectancy outcomes. *J Clin Oncol* 1993;11:777–782.

58. Gelber, R. D., et al. Quality-of-life adjusted evaluation of adjuvant therapies for operable breast cancer. *Ann Intern Med* 1991;114:621–8.

59. Tannock, I. Adjuvant therapy for node-negative breast cancer. *N Engl J Med* 1989;321:471–2 [letter].

60. McGuire, W. L., and G. M. Clark. Prognostic factors and treatment decisions in axillary-node-negative breast cancer. *N Engl J Med* 1992;326:1756–61 [review].

61. Early Breast Cancer Trialists' Collaborative Group. Systemic treatment of early breast cancer by hormonal, cytotoxic, or immune therapy. *Lancet* 1992;339:1–15, 71–85.

62. Ovarian ablation in early breast cancer: phoenix arisen? *Lancet* 1992;339:95–6 [editorial].

63. Charlson, M. E., and A. R. Feinstein. Rapid growth rate in breast cancer. *Lancet* 1982;i:1343–5.

64. Early Breast Cancer Trialists' Collaborative Group. Systemic treatment of early breast cancer by hormonal, cytotoxic, or immune therapy. *Lancet* 1992;339:1–15, 71–85.

65. Richards, M. A., et al. Adjuvant cyclophosphamide, methotrexate, and fluorouracil in patients with axillary node-positive breast cancer: an update of the Guy's/Manchester trial. *J Clin Oncol* 1990;8:2032–9.

66. Ovarian ablation in early breast cancer: phoenix arisen? *Lancet* 1992;339:95–6 [editorial].

67. Early Breast Cancer Trialists' Collaborative Group. Systemic treatment of early breast cancer by hormonal, cytotoxic, or immune therapy. *Lancet* 1992;339:1–15, 71–85.

68. Adjuvant systemic therapy for early breast cancer. *Lancet* 1992;339:27 [editorial].

69. Scottish Cancer Trials Breast Group and ICRF Breast Unit, Guy's Hospital, London. Adjuvant ovarian ablation versus CMF chemotherapy in premenopausal women with pathological stage II breast carcinoma: the Scottish trial. *Lancet* 1993;341:1293–8.

70. Fisher, B., et al. Ten-year results from the National Surgical Adjuvant Breast and Bowel Project (NSABP) clinical trial evaluating the use of L-phenylalanine mustard (L-PAM) in the management of primary breast cancer. *J Clin Oncol* 1986;4:929–41.

71. Ovarian ablation in early breast cancer: phoenix arisen? *Lancet* 1992;339:95–6 [editorial].

72. Bonadonna, G., et al. Adjuvant and neoadjuvant treatment of breast cancer with chemotherapy and/or endocrine therapy. *Semin Oncol* 1991;18:515–24.

73. Boccardo, F., et al. Chemotherapy versus tamoxifen versus chemotherapy plus tamoxifen in node-positive, estrogen receptor-positive breast cancer patients: results of a multicentric Italian study. *J Clin Oncol* 1990;8:1310–20.

74. Early Breast Cancer Trialists Collaborative Group. Systemic treatment of early breast cancer by hormonal, cytotoxic, or immune therapy. *Lancet* 1992;339:1–15, 71–85.

75. Bonadonna, G., et al. Primary chemotherapy to avoid mastectomy in tumors with diameters of three centimeters or more. *J Natl Cancer Inst* 1990;82:1539–45.

76. Bonadonna, G., et al. Adjuvant and neoadjuvant treatment of breast cancer with chemotherapy and/or endocrine therapy. *Semin Oncol* 1991;18:515–24.

77. Mittra, I. Has adjuvant treatment of breast cancer had an unfair trial? *BMJ* 1990;301:1317–9.

78. Epstein, S. S. *The politics of cancer*. Anchor Press/Doubleday, Garden City, NY, 1979, pp. 327, 456–7.

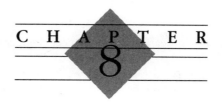

C H A P T E R
8

Why I Didn't Have Chemotherapy

CATHY

Deciding whether or not to do chemo is necessarily a personal choice. It should be based on both the specifics of your diagnosis (see Chapter 7) and who you are. It's important you feel free to make your own decision because your choice can so powerfully affect your life. Don't feel coerced by your doctor, family, friends, or even by what you read here.

I'd often thought about chemotherapy prior to my diagnosis. I'd known people with cancer and had been exposed to the usual media coverage of the subject. It's my belief that one day society will look back on the "chemotherapy era" the way we now look back on the bloodletting and leeching period of medical history — as primitive and barbaric.

Gilda Radner's *It's Always Something* helped me understand what chemotherapy can be like. Her book about her fight with ovarian cancer is unique. It's an unvarnished tale — without the whitewash so often applied by mainstream medicine and even by some breast cancer patients in their books. Although she clearly believed in her treatment and expected to get well, she graphically described the horrible side effects that chemo produced. Gilda's description of beginning treatment made my skin crawl.

> I would have to go into the hospital for two nights. The drugs would be administered intravenously. . . . Cytoxan is given to increase the effectiveness of cisplatin. . . . It can make the patient violently ill so doctors have learned that it is helpful to calm the patient with sleeping medications and steroids to avoid violent reactions.[1]

Whenever drugs with side effects are needed to mask the side effects of other drugs, I get nervous. I've had many reactions to prescription medications that were often not anticipated by medical doctors, so I have sound reason to be leery of drugs.

Gilda Radner did too. After writing about the nausea, she describes other side effects.

> A few mornings later, I woke up and the first thing my eyes focused on was hairs all over my pillowcase. . . . Looking down onto the bathtub floor while I was shampooing, I saw it was covered with hair swirling toward the drain — my hair. I was devastated.[2]

I totally identified with her feeling. I think most women can. Losing my hair, eyebrows, and eyelashes would have been a tremendous psychological shock at a time when my system was already overloaded. Chemo combinations for breast cancer may be less toxic than are ovarian cancer treatments, but severe side effects are still common.

I was appalled at what Radner suffered as a result of conventional medicine. It's not that she died; obviously, there are no guarantees. It's what she went through. I felt that in the name of modern medicine, Gilda Radner was put into a torture chamber more diabolical than anything dreamt up during the Inquisition. Nevertheless, I was well enough acquainted with the research to know that some types of cancer, like Hodgkin's disease and childhood leukemia, are often cured with chemotherapy. If I had had such a diagnosis, even with my strong negative feelings about chemo, I would have seriously considered it.

For many breast cancer patients, however, the outcome of chemo is not so impressive. For stage I, most women don't need or benefit from chemo (see Chapter 7). The very small chance of gaining an advantage didn't seem impressive enough to me to risk headaches, insomnia, low energy, diarrhea, malaise, ulcerations of the mouth, nausea, impaired immunity, depression, hair loss, weight gain, sexual dysfunction, loss of identity, early menopause, bleeding inflammation of the bladder, leukemia, lymphoma, and other complications that chemotherapy might entail.

I was most concerned with how chemo's potential side effects might alter my sense of identity and my ability to see myself as whole and healthy. The diagnosis alone was already taking its toll in that regard. Several well-meaning friends and family had compounded the problem by saying, "What, you're not still working, are you?" I felt they were seeing me with one foot in the grave. It was hard not to see myself that way. Adding the burden of severe side effects from chemotherapy was more than my psyche could bear. By choosing to avoid chemo, I was better able to put the pieces of my fragmented psyche back together. And, I didn't miss a day of work because of treatment. Continuing my usual work and relaxation routine was my personal statement of hope as well as a way to normalize a crazy-making situation.

Two physical factors also led me away from chemo. First, I have a slow recovery rate. As children, my brother and I got tonsillitis together almost yearly. I would stay in bed and do everything Mom said because I wanted to get back to school, while John ran around and did whatever he wanted. He beat me back to class every time. Later, as an adult, I once took two months to recuperate from a reaction to antibiotics.

I also have a low pain threshold. The dentist has to give me extra novocaine. Steve calls me "the Princess and the Pea" — one grain of sand in bed will keep me up all night. I can feel sunburn before people can see it. For these reasons, I didn't believe I would tolerate chemotherapy well.

Of every ten stage I women, seven will be cured without chemotherapy. For those seven, chemo can only make them sick. At least two out of the remaining three will die even if they take chemotherapy. I needed to find other choices.

Whatever your own decisions turn out to be, it is vital that you feel comfortable with them. A growing body of evidence suggests that your attitude may be critical to the outcome.[3] (See Chapters 10 and 11.) Bernie Siegel states it succinctly in *Love, Medicine, and Miracles:* "The most important thing is to pick a therapy that you believe in and proceed with a positive attitude."[4]

References

1. Radner G. *It's Always Something.* Simon and Schuster, New York, 1989, pp. 110–11.
2. Radner G. *It's Always Something.* Simon and Schuster, New York, 1989, p. 114.
3. Greer S., et al. Psychological response to breast cancer and 15-year outcome. *Lancet* 1990;335:49–50.
4. Siegel B. *Love, Medicine, and Miracles.* Harper & Row, New York, 1986, p. 129.

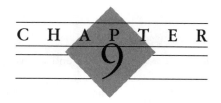

Tamoxifen

STEVE

The drug tamoxifen has nothing to do with chemotherapy. It doesn't kill cancer cells. It doesn't kill healthy cells. Tamoxifen's actions are complex, as is an understanding of who it helps and why. Nonetheless, there are some simple punch lines:

- Postmenopausal women who are ER-positive (have a positive estrogen receptor status) get the most benefit from tamoxifen.
- For postmenopausal women who are ER-negative, the benefits appear to outweigh the risks.
- For premenopausal women who are ER-positive, it's a tough call. Potential benefits are small.
- Premenopausal women who are ER-negative receive virtually no benefit.
- Tamoxifen is more effective in women who have cancer in their lymph nodes than in those whose nodes are cancer-free.
- Despite what you've heard, this drug has side effects. Sometimes they are serious.

Many breast cancer patients are offered tamoxifen (also called Nolvadex). It was developed more than 20 years ago, initially as a birth control pill. Tamoxifen didn't work as a contraceptive, but it was found to lower mammary cancer rates in animals. This discovery provided the impetus to study its effects in treating breast cancer.

WHAT DOES TAMOXIFEN DO?

The female hormone estrogen promotes the growth of breast cancer. In order to have any effect, estrogen must bind to special receptors in cells. Tamoxifen blocks these estrogen receptors (ERs), at least in breast cancer cells. In this way, tamoxifen interferes with estrogen. This is also the reason that ERs are measured during diagnosis; women with lots of ERs do better on tamoxifen.

Some side effects of tamoxifen demonstrate this anti-estrogenic effect. When women go through menopause, the hot flashes they experience result from decreased estrogen. Patients taking tamoxifen frequently have the same problem, reinforcing the notion that tamoxifen is basically anti-estrogenic.

The hypothesis that tamoxifen was simply an ER-blocking agent began to fall apart rather quickly, however. In theory, it might have worked better for premenopausal women because they have more estrogen to block than do women who are postmenopausal. However, the opposite is true: The anticancer effect of the drug is considerably more powerful in postmenopausal women. Researchers began to realize that the effects of tamoxifen are complicated.

The simplistic view of tamoxifen as an ER-blocker has suffered even more blows. Although the drug interferes with estrogen in the breast, it does the exact opposite in several other parts of the body, as we see later in this chapter. In other words, tamoxifen has both pro- and anti-estrogenic activity. It all depends on which part of the body we observe. If you're thinking ahead, you might have concerns that the pro-estrogenic effects might increase cancer risks in other organs. So do the researchers. I'll say more about this later.

Through years of investigation, scientists have begun to understand the complexities of tamoxifen. It turns out to be working at several different levels, each of which might be fighting cancer. Let's look at a few.

Tamoxifen increases a substance called sex hormone binding globulin, which in turn inactivates estrogen.[1] This effect is independent of estrogen blocking, suggesting that even women

with a low number of ERs may still be helped somewhat by tamoxifen. As we shall see, the research supports this idea.

Tamoxifen has also been found to decrease insulin-like
growth factor, a substance that stimulates the growth of breast
cancer cells;[2] this anticancer effect of tamoxifen is probably independent of estrogen. So is another recently discovered anticancer
effect of the drug — increasing a potent breast cancer growth inhibitor.[3] Tamoxifen can also reduce TGF-α — a substance that increases tumor growth;[4] while this effect happens only in women
with a sizable number of ERs, it may be unrelated to the estrogen-
blocking influence of the drug. Researchers are now wondering
how much of the therapeutic effect of tamoxifen has to do with
estrogen blocking and how much of it does not.

For years, the scientific community has known that patients
with a high number of ERs have improved chances of survival,
whether or not they take tamoxifen. This is paradoxical because
receptivity to estrogen, which is cancer-promoting, should make
the cancer grow faster. For some reason, it doesn't.

As researchers learned more about tamoxifen, more problems began to surface. It was discovered that the drug actually increases levels of estrogen.[5] Perhaps this is the body's way of com-
pensating for tamoxifen's blocking of ERs. Theoretically, an
increase in estrogen should make breast cancer more likely — not
less. And, in fact, tamoxifen has on occasion seemed to cause
breast cancer growth to accelerate.

You can begin to see how complicated the tamoxifen story has
become. Fortunately, while laboratory researchers are still developing an understanding of how the drug works, clinical studies are
providing much useful information. "Clinical" information refers to
what actually happens to the health of women who take the drug.

Clinical information can be more important than understanding how a drug works. We used aspirin to reduce inflammation
for many decades before we had any idea why it worked. For
centuries, we had no understanding of how medicinal plants
worked; knowledge was limited mostly to efficacy and toxicity.
Ultimately, clinical information is the most important thing we
need to know about tamoxifen as well.

To summarize, tamoxifen:

- Blocks estrogen activity in the breast
- Has anticancer properties independent of estrogen
- Affects the breast and other parts of the body in different ways; it sometimes has a pro-estrogenic effect
- Is better understood in terms of its clinical effects than its biochemical action

USING TAMOXIFEN TO TREAT BREAST CANCER

Now that thousands of breast cancer patients have been given tamoxifen, the overall results look good.* In 1992, the *Lancet* published a review of many studies; 30,000 of the breast cancer patients were randomly assigned to either take tamoxifen or not.[6]

The average patient in this collaborative report was followed for between five and six years. Of the patients taking tamoxifen, 74.4 percent survived, as compared with 70.9 percent in the no-tamoxifen group. These numbers mean that 744 lived for every 1,000 patients who received tamoxifen and 709 women lived for every 1,000 who did not get the drug. Thus, 35 additional women lived for every 1,000 women taking tamoxifen compared with those not taking it.

Through complex statistics, the authors called this a 17 percent reduction in "proportional annual risk." But clearly, only 3.5 percent of the women were helped by the drug during this period of time. (For the much smaller group followed for more than ten years, the 3.5 percent jumped to 6.2 percent.)

It's only human for researchers to sometimes couch their numbers in optimistic terms. If they think a drug is useful, they want to encourage doctors to use it. You may also wish to view the numbers in a positive light. It's important to understand,

---

*Unless otherwise stated, all trials discussed in this chapter deal with women previously treated with either lumpectomy (usually with radiation) or mastectomy.

however, that survival was not affected by tamoxifen for the vast majority of patients.

"Survival" tells us how many people are alive. Survival includes both those who are disease-free and those who have suffered a recurrence but are alive. The increase in survival brought about by tamoxifen (the 35 women for every 1,000) was accompanied by a much larger increase in "disease-free survival" — those women who hadn't had a recurrence.

In this same giant analysis, a total of 66.4 percent remained disease-free in the tamoxifen group. Only 59.9 percent of patients were disease-free in the no-tamoxifen group. (These figures reflect approximately five years of follow-up). So out of every 1,000 women, 65 more were spared a recurrence in the tamoxifen group than in the group not taking it.

Although you may be encouraged or discouraged by these overall numbers, they probably have little to do with your specific situation. You are not an "overall" statistic. And more detailed information is available for women who are ER-positive (meaning they have a relatively high number of estrogen receptors) than for women who are ER-negative. We also have more specific information about tamoxifen's effects in postmenopausal versus premenopausal women, as well as in node-negative versus node-positive patients. All these distinctions have a great impact on whether tamoxifen might help you. If you are a diagnosed breast cancer patient, you probably know which category you fit into in each case. Let's now look at how these various distinctions change the efficacy of tamoxifen.

ESTROGEN RECEPTOR STATUS

When breast cancer is biopsied or surgically removed, the laboratory measures the level of estrogen receptors in the cancerous tissue. The measurement is made in femtomoles per milligram (abbreviated fmol/mg), an exceedingly small amount.

In general, 10 fmol/mg is considered ER-positive and less than 10 ER-negative. However, some labs consider tumors ER-negative if under 3 fmol/mg and ER-positive if over 10 fmol/mg, leaving a fuzzy area in between. It gets even more confusing.

Some studies use as few as 2 fmol/mg as the cutoff point between ER-positive and ER-negative,[7] while others find 100 fmol/mg to be a more meaningful cutoff point.[8,9] Therefore, the label "ER-positive" means different things in different research articles. This variance makes it difficult to evaluate how the ER research relates to you. Nonetheless, the higher your ER number, the more you may assume that studies reporting results for ER-positive patients apply to you. And numbers well above 100 are not uncommon.

Most reports find that women who are ER-positive get better results with tamoxifen than do those who are ER-negative, regardless of menopausal status. Scientists reason that if you have more estrogen receptors to block, then blocking them should result in a more therapeutic effect. In fact, some studies find no therapeutic effect in ER-negative patients.[10,11]

The large *Lancet* collaborative report found ER-negative patients had absolutely no benefit from taking tamoxifen if they were premenopausal.[12] In general, as expected, ER-positive patients did better on tamoxifen regardless of their menopausal status. Also, postmenopausal women did better on tamoxifen even if they were ER-negative. In other words, the drug helped everyone except premenopausal, ER-negative women. If you fit both of these categories, taking tamoxifen appears to be a wasted effort.

The *Lancet* reported that the group helped most consisted of postmenopausal women with positive-ER status. For every four women in this group who died without the drug, one life was saved in the tamoxifen group. This is an impressive statistic for a drug lacking the extreme toxicity of chemotherapy.

A few doctors are recommending tamoxifen to almost all breast cancer patients. However, if you are premenopausal and had an ER-negative tumor, the therapeutic effects appear too small to justify taking the drug. Keep in mind, even though tamoxifen isn't nearly as dangerous as chemotherapy for most patients, it has side effects, and occasionally they may be serious (see "Tamoxifen Toxicity" later in this chapter).

If tamoxifen were to receive grades for its level of efficacy on the basis of ER and menopausal status, those marks would be:

- Postmenopausal with an ER-positive tumor: A
- Postmenopausal with an ER-negative tumor: B
- Premenopausal with an ER-positive tumor: C+
- Premenopausal with an ER-negative tumor: F

TAMOXIFEN AND NODE-NEGATIVE PATIENTS

You will recall that we are confining our comments to the treatment of early-stage patients only. "Early stage" generally means stage I and II. As a reminder, if you have no cancer in your lymph nodes and the tumor was 2 cm (0.8 inches) or smaller, you are considered stage I. If the tumor was larger, if limited cancer was found in lymph nodes, or both, you are generally considered stage II. Both stage I and II patients have no cancer in any distant part of their body (like liver or bone) and neither has extensive lymph node involvement. If your lymph nodes were sampled or dissected (see Chapter 3), your surgeon will be able to tell you what stage the cancer is.

In general, tamoxifen has been found to be more effective in helping node-positive patients than node-negative, although it appears to be useful in treating both. The *Lancet* collaborative trial looked at patients who had no cancer in their lymph nodes. Of those followed for more than ten years, about 75 percent survived with tamoxifen versus about 70 percent without it.[13]

Disease-free survival numbers were 68 percent for the node-negative tamoxifen group versus 63 percent for the node-negative control group. The difference between these two numbers means that one woman in 20 was kept disease-free by the drug. Tamoxifen was better at keeping women completely disease-free than in just keeping them alive, although both figures were improved. If you are postmenopausal, ER-positive, or both, your chances of being helped by tamoxifen would be better than the numbers given here, which apply to all node-negative women.

The American Medical Association has looked at several of the tamoxifen trials in node-negative women.[14] Some of the individual node-negative trials they reviewed obtained better results than the overall *Lancet* results, but the pattern was the same. Postmenopausal patients were helped more than premenopausal patients, and disease-free survival improved more than overall survival.

Some studies find absolutely no survival advantage in node-negative women taking tamoxifen, even if they had positive ER status.[15] Perhaps these women weren't followed long enough. Even in these trials, there was usually some improvement in disease-free survival.

If tamoxifen were to receive grades on its level of efficacy in *node-negative* women, those marks might be:

- Postmenopausal, ER-positive: B
- Postmenopausal, ER-negative: C
- Premenopausal, ER-positive: D
- Premenopausal, ER-negative: F

Although tamoxifen may not be as effective for stage I women as for women who have positive nodes, keep in mind that those of you with no cancer in your lymph nodes have a very good overall prognosis. And if you are postmenopausal, tamoxifen may still be worth considering.

TAMOXIFEN AND NODE-POSITIVE PATIENTS

Obviously, it's not good news to have cancer in your lymph nodes. However, if you are node-positive, tamoxifen works better. The *Lancet* analysis found that 50.4 percent of node-positive patients taking tamoxifen were alive after ten years, compared with only 42.4 percent of those not offered the drug.[16] Figures were equally impressive for disease-free survival. Trials looking at node-positive patients who are premenopausal versus those who are postmenopausal have found good results for both groups.[17]

Therefore, if you are a node-positive (stage II) patient, tamoxifen should definitely be discussed with your medical doctor, even when other indicators don't suggest tamoxifen usage. And tamoxifen appears useful in treating node-positive women who are also taking chemotherapy.

TAMOXIFEN AND MENOPAUSAL STATUS

In several places I've said that postmenopausal women generally get better results with tamoxifen than do premenopausal women. In fact, in 1988 the *New England Journal of Medicine* published an overview of 28 randomized tamoxifen trials and reported absolutely no improvement in survival for premenopausal women.[18,*] Years later, the giant *Lancet* overview extended the original *New England Journal* study and found that tamoxifen saved approximately one life for every 100 premenopausal patients put on the drug.[19] Again, disease-free survival was affected more than overall survival, and patients with positive nodes were helped more than node-negative patients.

Postmenopausal women fared better. About one life was saved for every twenty patients taking the drug.[20] If we focus on remaining disease-free, one out of every twelve postmenopausal patients taking the drug was spared a cancer recurrence.

Tamoxifen has proven sufficiently effective in treating postmenopausal women that some English researchers have actually tried it as the sole therapy.[21] That means patients weren't even treated surgically! Unfortunately for these women, the chance of breast cancer returning without surgery proved to be too high.[22] If, however, surgery is out of the question for you, due to

---

*For the sake of simplicity, most of the research divides women by age rather than by actual menopausal status. Therefore, in our discussion of the tamoxifen research, when we use the term *premenopausal,* it technically refers to women under 50 and *postmenopausal* refers to women beyond their 50th birthday. It's most likely, however, that the difference in efficacy between the two groups results from differing menopausal status and not a function of becoming 50 years old.

another debilitating disease or advanced age, tamoxifen should be considered because tamoxifen without surgery increases your chances of survival compared with no conventional treatment at all.[23]

Let's focus on two of the trials studied in the *New England Journal* compilation. The Danish and Scottish trials looked at postmenopausal patients having a combination of positive nodes and very high (over 100 fmol/mg) ER levels.[24] Remember, these three indicators suggest that tamoxifen will be unusually effective. As expected, both trials found tamoxifen very effective.* However, when patients with lower ER numbers were studied, the results were much less impressive.

Looking at only node-positive postmenopausal women, tamoxifen has substantially increased life expectancy and reduced the chance of getting breast cancer in the opposite breast, while increasing the average disease-free survival regardless of ER status.[25]

To review, if you are postmenopausal, your chances of being helped by tamoxifen are good. In fact, tamoxifen may be worth a try regardless of other details regarding your disease, though its chances of making a real difference increase significantly if you have a high number of ERs and/or are node-positive. If you are premenopausal, many, but not all, trials find it useless.

TAMOXIFEN TOXICITY

Oncologists generally consider tamoxifen a drug with few side effects; this is undoubtedly true when tamoxifen is compared with chemotherapy. However, tamoxifen *does* have side effects, and it's important not to gloss over problems that can result from taking it.

---

*The Danish trial reported 82 percent survival with tamoxifen and 61 percent without it. The Scottish trial reported 91 percent of those taking tamoxifen lived compared with only 55 percent of those who didn't.

Menopausal Symptoms

About half the women put on tamoxifen experience the hot flashes of menopause. Vaginal dryness and discharge are also common, though somewhat less so.

Menstrual Irregularity

Menstrual irregularity frequently occurs in premenopausal women on tamoxifen. Amenorrhea (absence of the menstrual cycle) often results from taking the drug. This effect can be permanent.

Because very little is known about how tamoxifen might affect the fetus, it is strongly recommended that birth control be used, though hormonal contraceptives are contraindicated because the estrogen they contain might interfere with the activity of tamoxifen.

Blood Clotting Disorders

Blood clotting disorders, which can be quite serious, occur in about 1 percent of patients taking tamoxifen.[26] Therefore, a history of thromboembolic (blood-clotting) disease makes you the wrong candidate for this drug.

Visual Impairment

Damage to the eyes has been reported in several trials. Decreased vision may be accompanied by damage to various parts of the visual apparatus. Most of the damage appears reversible when patients stop taking tamoxifen. At first, it was thought this side effect was rare, but a recent trial found that even low-dose tamoxifen caused ocular toxicity in more than 6 percent of the patients studied.[27] Anyone taking tamoxifen needs regular checkups with an ophthalmologist.

Uterine Cancer

As of 1993, approximately 70 cases of tamoxifen-linked endometrial (uterine) cancer have surfaced.[28] Evidence is mounting that breast cancer patients who take tamoxifen for more than two years (as currently prescribed) have well over twice the risk of endometrial cancer than do breast cancer patients not taking the drug.[29] Apparently, tamoxifen has a pro-estrogenic effect on the uterus even though it has the opposite effect on the breast.

Years ago when estrogen (Premarin) was first given to menopausal women to reduce hot flashes, a large increase in endometrial cancer resulted; but most cases of estrogen-induced endometrial cancer were not life-threatening. Most medical doctors have assumed that tamoxifen-induced endometrial cancer would also be fairly tame. But researchers from Yale University School of Medicine have found the opposite.[30] They claim, "it appears that women receiving tamoxifen as treatment for breast cancer who subsequently develop uterine cancer are at risk for high-grade endometrial cancers that have a poor prognosis."

The relatively small increase in the rate of endometrial cancer (which varies from study to study) is not as important as the larger reduction in breast cancer recurrence rates for those women most likely to benefit from tamoxifen. If you are unlikely to benefit, however, this potential toxicity must be weighed carefully.

Liver Cancer

Liver cancer has also been a concern among tamoxifen researchers. The drug is a powerful liver carcinogen in rats.[31,32] Typically, whatever causes cancer in animals does so in people as well. But, of the tens of thousands of women who have taken tamoxifen, only two cases of liver cancer have surfaced so far. Both women were taking 40 mg of tamoxifen per day — twice the usual dose.[33] Many medical doctors believe, therefore, that the liver cancer scare from rat studies will not haunt women taking the drug.

Nevertheless, Great Britain's Medical Research Council (MRC) withdrew its support from the primary prevention trial (where tamoxifen will be given to healthy women at high risk for breast cancer). Part of their concern was the possibility of inducing liver cancer in tamoxifen-treated women.[34] MRC's Secretary, Dai Rees, notes that most women in the tamoxifen trials have been followed for five to seven years or less — less time than it generally takes for liver cancer to surface after initial exposure to causative agents.[35]

It has also been suggested that increased rates of liver cancer could easily be overlooked. When liver cancer is discovered in breast cancer patients, it's usually assumed to have metastasized from the breast. Gary Williams, the medical director of the American Health Foundation, was quoted by *Science News* as saying, "I've specifically asked clinicians if a woman receiving tamoxifen has a liver mass, will they work her up to see if it is a liver cancer versus a metastasis from the breast . . . and the answer has always been 'No, we assume it's a metastasis.'"[36] In addition, liver failure unrelated to liver cancer has been reported for patients taking tamoxifen. So far, four deaths have resulted.[37]

If the apprehension about liver cancer turns out to be real, the increased risk will probably take years to show up and may affect only a few women. Nonetheless, the potential threat of liver cancer should give pause for thought. *Unlike breast cancer, liver cancer is almost invariably fatal.* As with the concern about endometrial cancer, however, this potential side effect needs to be weighed against the possible benefit from taking tamoxifen.

Psychological Symptoms

Depression has been reported as a potential side effect of tamoxifen.[38] The onset of the depression can be insidious; moreover, a breast cancer diagnosis itself can give you reason to be depressed. Therefore, it may be hard to tell whether it's the tamoxifen that's dragging you down. Individual cases of patients reporting an inability to concentrate have also appeared. If you take tamoxifen, carefully observe your mood and mental state. If you feel that the drug is causing depression or a lack of concentration, you might well be right. If the effect is strong enough, contact the prescribing physician and discuss a trial period of tamoxifen avoidance.

Asthma

Finally, as with several other drugs, inhalants, and even foods and food additives, tamoxifen can apparently trigger asthma attacks in some sensitive patients.[39]

POTENTIAL SIDE BENEFITS OF TAMOXIFEN

Surprisingly, tamoxifen has been reported to potentially reduce the risk of several conditions. None has been proven, but all are worth looking at.

Reduced Risk of Contralateral Breast Cancer

Breast cancer patients are at high risk for contracting cancer of the opposite (contralateral) breast. Swedish researchers reported an 8 percent risk of contralateral breast cancer in a ten-year follow-up of women with a previous breast cancer diagnosis.[40] Tamoxifen reduced this number to 5 percent. Most studies have reported similar reductions in contralateral breast cancer when patients are given tamoxifen.[41] However, this protective effect may not exist if the tamoxifen is taken for less than two years.[42] The reduction in contralateral risk has provided the major impetus for the new trials, which are using tamoxifen treatment in healthy women in order to prevent breast cancer (see "Tamoxifen and Healthy Women" later in this chapter).

Increased Bone Mass

Estrogen protects against bone loss, and interference with estrogen (for example, surgical removal of the ovaries in premenopausal women) leads to an increased risk of osteoporosis. For this reason, estrogen is frequently prescribed to protect women going through menopause from excessive bone loss. Because tamoxifen has anti-estrogenic effects in the breast, it was feared that it might induce osteoporosis.

Fortunately, it has been found that tamoxifen does not appear to adversely affect bone.[43,44] In fact, lumbar (lower back) bone density has actually been reported to increase as a result of taking the drug.[45] Apparently, tamoxifen may have a pro-estrogenic effect on at least one type of bone.

Increases in bone density sound promising but are not the final word regarding bone health. In the last few years researchers found that supplemental fluoride increases bone density but also increases fracture rates. In other words, while increased bone mass sounds good, we need to make sure the additional bone is normal, healthy, and strong. The best way to assess this issue is to look at fracture rates. When fracture rates decline as a result of an intervention (such as exercise or calcium supplementation), we know we've done the right thing. As yet there are not enough data to tell us whether tamoxifen will actually reduce fracture rates. What researchers are now hoping for is a drop in vertebral (spinal) fracture rates with at least no negative effect on hip fracture rates.

Heart Disease Prevention

In addition to protecting bones, estrogen also reduces the risk of heart disease. Therefore, it was feared that tamoxifen might increase cardiovascular death rates by interfering with estrogen. And the average woman is already much more likely to die from heart disease than from breast cancer.

Instead, tamoxifen lowers serum cholesterol levels substantially.[46,47] The drop is primarily in the LDL fraction, the portion of cholesterol associated with heart disease. The Scottish trial using tamoxifen to treat breast cancer has also reported a decrease in cardiovascular death rates.[48] This has recently been confirmed by Swedish researchers.[49] Virtually any drug that reduces serum LDL cholesterol levels will reduce the risk of heart attacks. And, while other prescription drugs used to lower cholesterol are frequently associated with an increase in other causes of death, this pattern has not been seen with tamoxifen. In other words, it's possible that tamoxifen may turn out to be a safer cholesterol-lowering drug than those drugs currently being used for that purpose.

TAMOXIFEN AND CHEMOTHERAPY

Until recently, most patients have been offered either chemotherapy or tamoxifen — not both. Some researchers were concerned the two therapies could cancel each other out. At least one trial has reported better results for tamoxifen alone than for chemotherapy plus tamoxifen in some patients.[50] (This trial was discussed in Chapter 7.)

Generally, medical doctors prescribe tamoxifen for postmenopausal patients and chemotherapy for premenopausal patients. The scientific support for this distinction has already been discussed in this chapter and Chapter 7. However, it now appears that chemo may marginally help some postmenopausal patients, and tamoxifen makes sense for some premenopausal patients with high levels of ERs. Therefore, several researchers are giving tamoxifen and chemo to the same patients.

Japanese researchers have looked at the effects of adding tamoxifen to chemotherapy in ER-positive patients.[51] Women with large tumors and negative nodes appeared to do better on chemo plus tamoxifen than on chemo alone, but other groups did not. American researchers have also looked at the possibility of adding tamoxifen to chemotherapy.[52] One group reported added benefits in the chemo-plus-tamoxifen group if women were postmenopausal, node-positive and ER-positive — in other words, the patients previously shown to benefit most from tamoxifen.

Perhaps the chemo-plus-tamoxifen trial receiving most attention in the United States has been the National Surgical Adjuvant Breast and Bowel Project (NSABP) protocol B-16.[53] This study focused on postmenopausal, node-positive women with tamoxifen-responsive tumors* — again, those women most likely to benefit from tamoxifen alone. The NSABP group reported that chemo-plus-tamoxifen worked significantly better than tamoxifen alone in

---

*Surprisingly, NSABP defines "tamoxifen-responsive" for women in their 50s as being progesterone receptor (PR) positive or at least 60 years of age regardless of receptor status.

these select women. At three years, the survival rate was 93 percent for women taking both treatments and 85 percent for the tamoxifen-only group. The chemo-plus-tamoxifen treatment resulted in 84 percent of the patients remaining totally disease-free, compared with only 67 percent for the tamoxifen-only group.[54] A later follow-up of this report showed similar results after an additional year.[55] As a result of this outcome, Bernard Fisher of the NSABP has begun to recommend that postmenopausal, node-positive, tamoxifen-responsive women take both chemotherapy and tamoxifen.

The large *Lancet* collaborative study combined the results of NSABP B-16 with many other trials. The *Lancet* also found better results with chemo and tamoxifen than with tamoxifen alone in preventing a recurrence, though there was no additional survival advantage.[56] They found that chemo and tamoxifen are better together than chemo alone for both survival and recurrence rates.

With the advent of NSABP B-16 and several other trials, some clinicians are considering both therapies for their postmenopausal patients. In fact, a recent conference of virtually all leading breast cancer researchers held at St. Gallen, Switzerland, recommended both treatments for all node-positive patients 70 years old or younger, unless they are both premenopausal and ER-negative.[57] For the moment, however, many practicing oncologists have been slow to use chemo and tamoxifen with the same patient—and for good reason. A review of the chemo-plus-tamoxifen trials up to 1991 found that for every study reporting good results, another reported that the combination is no better than tamoxifen alone.[58] And suffering the side effects of chemotherapy unnecessarily would be tragic.

Available information regarding the combination of chemo and tamoxifen is increasing rapidly; but at least for now, using this combination still seems somewhat questionable.

TAMOXIFEN AND HEALTHY WOMEN: THE PREVENTION TRIAL

Recently, the Breast Cancer Prevention Trial, which is in progress, has received much press coverage. This trial is studying women who have never had breast cancer to see if tamoxifen can prevent the disease from ever occurring. This is called "primary prevention." (Preventing a recurrence is called "secondary prevention.")

If you are not a breast cancer patient but are reading this book to reduce your chances of getting the disease, this section should be of interest to you. If you are a breast cancer patient, you may want to know about tamoxifen and primary prevention for the sake of your daughters and sisters who, as you probably know, are at higher than normal risk.

As long ago as January 1986, English researchers suggested that tamoxifen should be used in healthy women who are at high risk for breast cancer.[59] As a result of that suggestion, the National Cancer Institute (NCI), in collaboration with NSABP, is now giving 16,000 women from the United States and Canada either tamoxifen or a placebo for five years at the cost of $68 million.

This trial is both special and controversial because it's the first time a drug with known (and probably unknown) side effects has been used in healthy people for the purpose of primary prevention. It's one thing to use a drug with associated risks when you're fighting a life-threatening disease; it's entirely another matter when drugs with potentially serious side effects are given to completely healthy women. The amount of risk people are willing to take under these circumstances should obviously be much lower.

However, many of the women in this study may not be fully aware of the risks involved. The House Subcommittee on Human Resources has discovered that most of the informed consent forms given to prospective participants in this trial contain one or more serious omissions of risk data.[60] Although this omission may just be an oversight, most participants have not been properly informed about potential side effects. Attempts are being made to solve this problem by revising the informed consent forms.

Proponents of the study are fixing this problem because they understand that participants need to be informed about all possible known risks. These proponents say the potential dangers of tamoxifen are acceptable because the women in this study are at very high risk of becoming breast cancer patients. But are they?

Any woman 60 years of age or more is considered by this study to be at high risk. Younger women with a risk as high as the average 60-year-old are also allowed into the study. At this level of risk, more than 98 percent of the patients are not expected to get breast cancer during the five-year trial, even if they are in the placebo group![61] Researchers hope that tamoxifen will be as effective in primary prevention as it has been in preventing contralateral breast cancer in women who are already breast cancer patients. But even if this were true, tamoxifen would prevent cancer in only between 0.7 and 1.6 percent of the women in the trial — in other words, in about 1 woman for every 100 taking the drug.[62] And some estimates of how many women might be helped are as low as 0.5 percent or 1 woman in 200.[63]

For premenopausal women, participating in the trial seems especially unreasonable. Some side effects (like menstrual irregularity) occur only in premenopausal women, yet the therapeutic track record of the drug is not as good for younger women. As mentioned earlier, the reduced risk of contralateral tumors in breast cancer patients has been a major incentive in getting this primary prevention trial off the ground. However, even this good news (reduced contralateral tumors) comes mostly from postmenopausal patients. Furthermore, some researchers are concerned that tamoxifen might breed drug-resistant tumors, an idea supported by some of the animal data.

Sam Epstein, a professor of occupational and environmental health at the University of Illinois School of Public Health, and Adriane Fugh-Berman, from the National Women's Health Network, have weighed the evidence and come down heavily in favor of stopping the trial.[64] Even the Food and Drug Administration Oncologic Drugs Advisory Committee recommended that approval be withheld until the study is limited to women at significantly higher risk.[65]

None of us has a crystal ball, and only the future will tell whether tamoxifen is worth considering for primary prevention. If I were a woman, however, I'd let someone else be in the first row of guinea pigs. If you are considering participation in the trial for yourself or someone you know, reread the section of this chapter dealing with side effects. Remember, even if the trial is a success, you stand about a 99 percent chance of not reaping the benefits. With odds like that, I don't take prescription drugs for prevention purposes, especially when the outcome is unknown.

Does participation in the trial make sense for anyone? Probably. By the time you're reading this, BRCA1, a gene that causes familial breast cancer, will probably have been isolated.[66] Typically, it is found in families where breast cancer is rampant. Once the gene is discovered, a blood test should rapidly become available to every woman. If you test positive for BRCA1, your lifetime chance of getting the disease is higher than 85 percent, and the need to take greater than normal risks to prevent the disease becomes obvious. That situation might make prophylactic tamoxifen a reasonable option. Discuss it with your doctors, being sure before the meeting that they are familiar with the research.[67,68,69]

Why tamoxifen instead of other means of primary prevention? Drugs are high-profit items, so there is much interest in exploring their potential. Who would benefit if a dietary/lifestyle program were successful, besides the women in the study and their families?

There is another reason that other forms of primary prevention have been put on the back burner. The conventional medical establishment has little interest and even less faith that such a program would be feasible. Consider what researchers from the National Institutes of Health (NIH) have to say:

> dietary intervention in the United States is limited by the relatively high level of saturated fat in the average American diet.[70]

This is precisely the reason that dietary intervention could reduce breast cancer risk in the United States: We have something to change, but conventional researchers believe that the average American woman is unwilling to change. Isn't that attitude a bit presumptuous? Who said you're average anyway? These NIH researchers go on to rationalize why diet couldn't or shouldn't be used to prevent breast cancer:

> Risk ratios for breast cancer between highest and lowest quintiles of saturated fat intake are less than twofold in most epidemiologic studies of

American women, and compliance with prescribed diets in prevention studies is variable.[71]

Statistically, "less than twofold" means that a dietary change might reduce a woman's risk by less than 50 percent. Nobody pushing the Breast Cancer Prevention Trial expects the tamoxifen to do nearly that well. And proof exists from several research groups (see Chapter 12) that good compliance is possible.

TAMOXIFEN CHECKLIST

If you decide to take tamoxifen, discuss the following checklist with the prescribing medical doctor:

1. There is clear evidence that better results are obtained if tamoxifen is taken for more than two years — preferably five.
2. Schedule regular visits with an ophthalmologist. Remember — tamoxifen can induce ocular damage.
3. If you are premenopausal, you should not be taking hormonal contraceptives because they might potentially interact with the tamoxifen.
4. Nonetheless, if you are premenopausal and taking tamoxifen, you must be on some form of birth control if you are heterosexually active. Effects of the drug on the human fetus are unknown.
5. To be vigilant in identifying side effects of the drug, have a yearly physical. Also watch for unexplained depression or poor concentration.
6. Don't take tamoxifen if you have had a history of thromboembolic disease or macular degeneration (an ocular condition).
7. Be prepared for menstruation to cease or become irregular.

References

1. Sakai, F., et al. Increases in steroid binding globulins induced by tamoxifen in patients with carcinoma of the breast. *J Endocrinol* 1978;76:219–26.
2. Pollack, M., et al. Effect of tamoxifen on serum insulinlike growth factor I levels in stage I breast cancer patients. *J Natl Cancer Inst* 1990;82:1693–7.

3. Butta, A., et al. Induction of transforming growth factor β_1, in human breast cancer *in vivo* following tamoxifen treatment. *Cancer Res* 1992;52:4261–4.

4. Noguchi, S., et al. Down-regulation of transforming growth factor-α by tamoxifen in human breast cancer. *Cancer* 1993;72:131–6.

5. Jordan, C. V. Long-term adjuvant tamoxifen: an appropriate chemosuppressive therapy for breast cancer. American Cancer Society's Thirty-second Science Writers' Seminar, Daytona Beach, Florida, March 28, 1990.

6. Early Breast Cancer Trialists' Collaborative Group. Systemic treatment of early breast cancer by hormonal, cytotoxic, or immune therapy. *Lancet* 1992;339:1–15,71–85.

7. Rutqvist, L. E., et al. Contralateral primary tumors in breast cancer patients in a randomized trial of adjuvant tamoxifen therapy. *J Natl Cancer Inst* 1991;83:1299–1306.

8. Rose, C., et al. Beneficial effect of adjuvant tamoxifen therapy in primary breast cancer patients with high oestrogen receptor values. *Lancet* 1985;i:16–19.

9. Stewart, H. J., and R. Prescott. Adjuvant tamoxifen therapy and receptor levels. *Lancet* 1985;i:573 [letter].

10. Rose, C., et al. Beneficial effect of adjuvant tamoxifen therapy in primary breast cancer patients with high oestrogen receptor values. *Lancet* 1985;i:16–19.

11. Stewart, H. J., and R. Prescott. Adjuvant tamoxifen therapy and receptor levels. *Lancet* 1985;i:573 [letter].

12. Early Breast Cancer Trialists' Collaborative Group. Systemic treatment of early breast cancer by hormonal, cytotoxic, or immune therapy. *Lancet* 1992;339:1–15,71–85.

13. Early Breast Cancer Trialists' Collaborative Group. Systemic treatment of early breast cancer by hormonal, cytotoxic, or immune therapy. *Lancet* 1992;339:1–15,71–85.

14. Council on Scientific Affairs, American Medical Association. Report of the council on scientific affairs: Management of patients with node-negative breast cancer. *Arch Intern Med* 1993;153:58–67.

15. Fisher, B., et al. A randomized clinical trial evaluating tamoxifen in the treatment of patients with node-negative breast cancer who have estrogen-receptor-positive tumors. *N Engl J Med* 1989;320:479–84.

16. Early Breast Cancer Trialists' Collaborative Group. Systemic treatment of early breast cancer by hormonal, cytotoxic, or immune therapy. *Lancet* 1992;339:1–15,71–85.

17. Nolvadex Adjuvant Trial Organisation. Controlled trial of tamoxifen as single adjuvant agent in management of early breast cancer. *Lancet* 1985;i:836–40.

18. Early Breast Cancer Trialists' Collaborative Group. Effects of adjuvant tamoxifen and of cytotoxic therapy on mortality in early breast cancer. *N Engl J Med* 1988;319:1681–92.

19. Early Breast Cancer Trialists' Collaborative Group. Systemic treatment of early breast cancer by hormonal, cytotoxic, or immune therapy. *Lancet* 1992;339:1–15,71–85.

20. Early Breast Cancer Trialists' Collaborative Group. Systemic treatment of early breast cancer by hormonal, cytotoxic, or immune therapy. *Lancet* 1992;339:1–15,71–85.

21. Dixon, J. M. Treatment of elderly patients with breast cancer — tamoxifen alone is no longer justified. *BMJ* 1992;304:996–7.

22. Rubens, R. D. Age and the treatment of breast cancer. *J Clin Oncol* 1993;11:3–4. [editorial].

23. Allan, S. G., et al. Tamoxifen as primary treatment of breast cancer in elderly or frail patients: a practical management. *BMJ* 1985;290:358.

24. Stewart, H. J., and R. Prescott. Adjuvant tamoxifen therapy and receptor levels. *Lancet* 1985;i:573 [letter].

25. Cummings, F. J. Adjuvant tamoxifen versus placebo in elderly women with node-positive breast cancer: long-term follow-up and causes of death. *J Clin Oncol* 1993;11:29–35.

26. Fisher, B., et al. A randomized clinical trial evaluating tamoxifen in the treatment of patients with node-negative breast cancer who have estrogen-receptor-positive tumors. *N Engl J Med* 1989;320:479–84.

27. Pavlidis, N. A., et al. Clear evidence that long-term, low-dose tamoxifen treatment can induce ocular toxicity. *Cancer* 1992;69:2961–4.

28. Seoud, M. A-F., J. Johson, and J. C. Weed, Jr. Gynecologic tumors in tamoxifen-treated women with breast cancer. *Obstet Gynecol* 1993;82:165–9.

29. van Leeuwen F. E., et. al. Risk of endometrial cancer after tamoxifen treatment of breast cancer. *Lancet* 1994;343:448–52.

30. Magriples, U., et al. High-grade endometrial carcinoma in tamoxifen-treated breast cancer patients. *J Clin Oncol* 1993;11:485–90.

31. Williams, G. M., et al. The triphenylethylene drug tamoxifen is a strong liver carcinogen in the rat. *Carcinogenesis* 1993;14:315–7.

32. Greaves, P., et al. Two-year carcinogenicity study of tamoxifen in Alderley Park wistar-derived rats. *Cancer Res* 1993;53:3919–24.

33. Fornander, T., et al. Adjuvant tamoxifen in early breast cancer: occurrence of new primary cancers. *Lancet* 1989;i:117–120.

34. Raloff, J. Tamoxifen quandary. *Sci News* 1992;141:266–9.

35. Raloff, J. Tamoxifen quandary. *Sci News* 1992;141:266–9.

36. Raloff, J. Tamoxifen quandary. *Sci News* 1992;141:266–9.

37. Ching, C. K., P. G. Smith, and R. G. Long. Tamoxifen-associated hepatocellular damage and agranulocytosis. *Lancet* 1992;339:940 [letter].

38. Nolvadex Adjuvant Trial Organisation. Controlled trial of tamoxifen as single adjuvant agent in management of early breast cancer. *Lancet* 1985;i:836–40.

39. Smith, R. P., et al. Tamoxifen-induced asthma. *Lancet* 1993;341:772 [letter].

40. Rutqvist, L. E., et al. Contralateral primary tumors in breast cancer patients in a randomized trial of adjuvant tamoxifen therapy. *J Natl Cancer Inst* 1991;83:1299–1306.

41. Early Breast Cancer Trialists' Collaborative Group. Systemic treatment of early breast cancer by hormonal, cytotoxic, or immune therapy. *Lancet* 1992;339:1–15,71–85.

42. Andersson, M., et al. Incidence of new primary cancer after adjuvant tamoxifen therapy and radiotherapy for early breast cancer. *J Natl Cancer Inst* 1991;83:1013–7.

43. Wright, C. D. P., et al. Effect of long term tamoxifen treatment on bone turnover in women with breast cancer. *BMJ* 1993;306:429–30.

44. Fornander, T., et al. Long-term adjuvant tamoxifen in early breast cancer: effect on bone mineral density in postmenopausal women. *J Clin Oncol* 1990;8:1019–24.

45. Love, R. R., et al. Effects of tamoxifen on bone mineral density in postmenopausal women with breast cancer. *N Engl J Med* 1992;326:852–6.

46. Dewar, J. A., et al. Long term effects of tamoxifen on blood lipid values in breast cancer. *BMJ* 1992;305:225–6.

47. Love, R. R., et al. Effects of tamoxifen on cardiovascular risk factors in postmenopausal women. *Ann Intern Med* 1991;115:860–4.

48. McDonald, C. C., and H. J. Stewart. Fatal myocardial infarction in the Scottish adjuvant tamoxifen trial. *BMJ* 1991;303:435–7.

49. Rutqvist, L. E., and A. Mattsson. Cardiac and thromboembolic morbidity among postmenopausal women with early-stage breast cancer in a randomized trial of adjuvant tamoxifen. *J Natl Cancer Inst* 1993; 1398–1406.

50. Boccardo, F., et al. Chemotherapy versus tamoxifen versus chemotherapy plus tamoxifen in node-positive, estrogen receptor-positive breast cancer patients: results of a multicentric Italian study. *J Clin Oncol* 1990; 8:1310–20.

51. Toi, M., et al. Randomized adjuvant trial to evaluate the addition of tamoxifen and PSK to chemotherapy in patients with primary breast cancer. *Cancer* 1992;70:2475–83.

52. Crowe, J. P., et al. Short-term tamoxifen plus chemotherapy: superior results in node-positive breast cancer. *Surgery* 1990;108:619–28.

53. Fisher, B., et al. Postoperative chemotherapy and tamoxifen compared with tamoxifen alone in the treatment of positive-node breast cancer patients aged 50 years and older with tumors responsive to tamoxifen: results from the National Surgical Adjuvant Breast and Bowel Project B-16. *J Clin Oncol* 1990;8:1005–18.

54. Fisher, B., et al. Postoperative chemotherapy and tamoxifen compared with tamoxifen alone in the treatment of positive-node breast cancer patients aged 50 years and older with tumors responsive to tamoxifen: results from the National Surgical Adjuvant Breast and Bowel Project B-16. *J Clin Oncol* 1990;8:1005–18.

55. Fisher, B. A biological perspective of breast cancer: contributions of the National Surgical Adjuvant Breast and Bowel Project clinical trials. *CA* 1991;41:97–111.

56. Early Breast Cancer Trialists' Collaborative Group. Systemic treatment of early breast cancer by hormonal, cytotoxic, or immune therapy. *Lancet* 1992;339:1–15,71–85.

57. Glick, J. H., et al. Meeting highlights: adjuvant therapy for primary breast cancer. *J Natl Cancer Inst* 1992;84:1479–85.

58. Bonadonna, G., et al. Adjuvant and neoadjuvant treatment of breast cancer with chemotherapy and/or endocrine therapy. *Seminars Oncol* 1991;18:515–24.

59. Cuzick, J., et al. The prevention of breast cancer. *Lancet* 1986;i:83–6.

60. Raloff, J. Tamoxifen and informed consent dissent. *Sci News* 1992; 142:378–80.

61. Raloff, J. Tamoxifen and informed consent dissent. *Sci News* 1992; 142:378–80.

62. Bluming, A. Z. Letter. *Lancet* 1993;341:694–5.

63. Fugh-Berman, A., and S. Epstein. Tamoxifen: disease prevention or disease substitution? *Lancet* 1992;340:1143–5.

64. Fugh-Berman, A., and S. Epstein. Tamoxifen: disease prevention or disease substitution? *Lancet* 1992;340:1143–5.

65. Raloff, J. Tamoxifen and informed consent dissent. *Sci News* 1992; 142:378–80.

66. Breo, D. L. Altered fates — counseling families with inherited breast cancer. *JAMA* 1993;269:2017–22.

67. Breo, D. L. Altered fates — counseling families with inherited breast cancer. *JAMA* 1993;269:2017–22.

68. King, M. C., et al. Inherited breast and ovarian cancer — what are the risks? What are the choices? *JAMA* 1993;269:1975–80.

69. Biesecker, B. B., et al. Genetic counseling for families with inherited susceptibility to breast and ovarian cancer. *JAMA* 1993;269:1970–4.

70. Nayfield, S. G., et al. Potential role of tamoxifen in prevention of breast cancer. *J Natl Cancer Inst* 1991;83:1450–9.

71. Nayfield, S. G., et al. Potential role of tamoxifen in prevention of breast cancer. *J Natl Cancer Inst* 1991;83:1450–9.

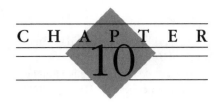

C H A P T E R
10

Your Alternative Choices for Treatment

STEVE

Medical doctors often say there's no *proof* that you can do anything to treat breast cancer through diet, vitamins, and herbs. This is essentially true; in fact, very little evidence exists one way or the other. (This is not true of prevention, however, as we shall see later.)

Few studies tell us that breast cancer can be treated with alternative therapies because not many people are studying them. Why not? It's like the old story of the drunkard who lost his keys down the block but looked for them under the lamp post because "that's where the light is." Except for a handful of studies, conventional researchers generally haven't looked for answers outside the realm of surgery, chemo, and radiation, even though solutions are not forthcoming from those therapies. Because the research community has studied alternatives so sporadically, it's most unlikely that positive or negative results could have been found.

The American Cancer Society (ACS) lists "Questionable Methods," which include many alternatives. In commentaries about these therapies, the ACS discredits them with innuendo, and makes them appear to be quackery. No doubt many of them are useless at best; but some may have value. Innuendo aside, what careful reading of the ACS statements reveals is that we often know very little about these therapies because they haven't been studied.

The ultimate effect of the ACS list is to make research funds unavailable for alternative cancer inquiry, thus creating a classic Catch-22. After a therapy is put on the ACS list, it rarely gets the

128

funding needed to prove itself. The ACS leadership thus shows that even though it knows little about alternative therapies, it has no interest in finding out more. Although much cancer research is not directly controlled by the ACS, most other funding institutions usually follow the ACS lead and don't support research that investigates "questionable methods." The new and highly publicized Office of Alternative Medicine at the National Institutes of Health is, in reality, a financial drop in the bucket, unlikely to change this situation in a meaningful way.[1]

To understand what may be the underlying causes of this failure to investigate alternative treatment, consider the consequences of a breakthrough in an alternative therapy. The publicity would be an embarrassment to conventional medicine, which frequently fails — in some cases, consistently. For example, pancreatic cancer, mesothelioma, and a variety of other cancers simply don't respond to conventional medicine; but even in such circumstances, patients are sent to the oncologist for treatment. This unquestioned monopoly would be challenged if solutions started to appear from nonconventional sources.

In the event of an alternative breakthrough, most cancer research institutions would have to regroup. They are now set up primarily to study surgery, chemotherapy, and radiation. Laboratories contain equipment designed for those therapies, and researchers have been trained to work with them. Practicing medical doctors might also have difficulty recommending successful alternative therapies; they're untrained in these areas and most are ideologically opposed to them. Even the basic philosophy of allopathic (conventional) medicine — "stop the symptom or destroy the disease" rather than "help the healing powers of the body to overcome the disease" — would be called into question by success arising from alternative research.

More troubling is the political connection: A well-documented review of the history of the National Cancer Institute (NCI) and ACS, the two largest funding organizations, shows that people in decision-making positions often represent the drug companies marketing chemotherapy or even the research institutes receiving NCI and ACS grant money.[2]

When evidence begins to suggest that a nonconventional therapy is useful, as is now the case with psychological intervention (see "Psychological Intervention," later in this chapter), the medical community has tended to ignore or discredit it. Ultimately, such an unconventional therapy risks being placed on the Questionable Methods list, thus limiting future funding.

Despite the lack of ACS/NCI-funded nonconventional research, a few clinical trials have been done with alternative approaches. Let's look.

METABOLIC THERAPY (LAETRILE)

One alternative approach that has been partially researched is "metabolic therapy," which centers on laetrile and includes vitamins, enzymes, and an altered diet. Laetrile is a variation of an isolate discovered in apricot pits by Ernst T. Krebs — father and son. Years ago, they proposed a theory suggesting that the cyanide in laetrile might selectively kill cancer cells.

The metabolic approach has been investigated by the Mayo Clinic, where researchers found that it doesn't help terminal cancer patients.[3] Although it has been argued that the "laetrile" in common use is different from the true Laetrile,[4] this doesn't change the fact that the Mayo Clinic did use what is typically available to cancer patients (although they looked only at late-stage patients).

The oldest and probably best known of the laetrile "metabolic" clinics is the Contreras Hospital in Tijuana, Mexico. A list of patients (complete with phone numbers and addresses) who were treated with apparent success by the metabolic approach is available from this facility. But we don't know how many patients were needed before these apparently successful cases could be amassed. Actual studies showing that laetrile "works" have been done only with animals to date and typically under conditions very different from the use of laetrile in humans.[5]* Therefore,

---

*A brief review of animal studies appears in Ralph Moss's *The Cancer Industry* (Paragon House, New York, 1991) pages 144–5, with a discussion of the politics of laetrile on pages 153–85.

there is as yet no research supporting the use of laetrile for breast cancer patients.

In 1983–84, three naturopathic doctors, Ellen Baumgartner Dale, Sharon DeKadt, and I, conducted a laetrile/metabolic therapy investigation independent of the medical establishment.[6] We interviewed consecutive patients as they began treatment at the Contreras Hospital. Our preliminary results confirmed what the Mayo Clinic researchers reported.[7] In a five-year follow-up, all twenty-two patients we followed died from a wide variety of malignancies, including breast cancer.[8] As with the Mayo Clinic study, these patients were late-stage. This strongly suggests that, in the absence of other data, it does not make sense to use the metabolic therapy to treat breast cancer, though admittedly nothing is known about the effects of such treatment with early-stage disease.

SHARK CARTILAGE

In 1985, a report on thirty-one cancer patients treated with bovine (cow) cartilage appeared in the medical literature.[9] Most of these patients had slim chances to begin with, but many fared remarkably well. Four breast cancer patients were in the group. At least three of the four had advanced disease when they began receiving the cartilage, administered by injections and orally. To varying degrees, all four appeared to be helped, though evaluation with such small numbers is difficult. In the years following the publication of this provocative article, most cancer researchers somehow forgot about cartilage.

Then in 1992–93, a book called *Sharks Don't Get Cancer*,[10] by Bill Lane and Linda Comac, and a *60 Minutes* TV show drew the public's attention to cartilage as a potential cancer treatment.

Sharks rarely do get cancer. Unlike most animals, the skeleton of the shark is made of cartilage, not bone. Different from other parts of the body, cartilage is basically "avascular" — it lacks blood vessels. Most cancers (including breast cancer) require a generous supply of blood in order to keep growing. Cancer cells are somehow able to direct the body to build new blood vessels to supply the tumor.

Scientists from M.I.T. have shown that shark cartilage contains substances that inhibit this process of vascularization[11] and they have begun to isolate these molecules.[12] Cartilage from other animals probably has a similar effect; but there's more cartilage in a shark, and some researchers believe shark cartilage is more effective than cartilage taken from bovine or other sources.

The basic concept of shark cartilage seems simple: If cancer needs a special blood supply and substances in the cartilage can impair the growth of new blood vessels, then perhaps shark cartilage can starve the tumor. European scientists have apparently shown that cancerous tumors in animals can be reduced in size by feeding them shark cartilage.[13] I say "apparently" because, to date, this information has only been reported secondhand; the researchers themselves have not yet published these data.

Years after our preliminary investigation of laetrile, the Contreras Hospital began to use shark cartilage to treat late-stage patients.[14] The cartilage was administered into the vagina and also as a retention enema.* Fifteen grams of powdered cartilage in a solution were used in each of the two administrations per day. Eight patients were in the study, and only one of them had breast cancer. They were followed for eleven weeks. Seven of the eight had substantial reduction in tumor size — all except the breast cancer patient. Long-term follow-up of these eight patients has not been published; but following the preliminary results, all eight were switched to a different product and did poorly.[15] Thus, we have no proof that the cartilage helped them in the long run.

Anecdotes of early-stage breast cancer patients using 7 grams per day of shark cartilage (taken orally) and having no recurrences appeared in both *Sharks Don't Get Cancer* and the Contreras Hospital research, but details were not provided. Keep

---

*In *Sharks Don't Get Cancer* (page 95), the authors claim, "Dr. Ernesto Contreras, Jr., had observed that when treating advanced cancer patients, enzymes and other nutrients are often more effective when given via retention enemas than when administered orally." As yet, however, absorption rates from different routes of administration (oral, rectal, vaginal, etc.) have simply not been researched.

in mind that many breast cancer patients survive disease-free for decades after conventional treatment, so these anecdotes prove nothing.

Although other doctors have also experimented with shark cartilage in the treatment of cancer, most of this work has not been published. Lane and Comar's book describes the work of Roscoe Van Zandt, a medical doctor in Arlington, Texas, who has also worked at the Hoxsey clinic (see "The Hoxsey Formula," later in this chapter). According to Lane and Comar, Van Zandt treated eight women with advanced breast cancer, giving them 30 to 60 grams per day of shark cartilage administered orally.[16] All eight had a reduction in tumor size within eight weeks. But these same women were also treated simultaneously with the Hoxsey treatment.[17] It's possible these patients were helped by the Hoxsey therapy. It therefore hasn't been proved that the shark cartilage was responsible for the tumor shrinkage. For the most part, the long-term outcome for these women is not known, though one died of causes unrelated to her cancer and at least one died from the breast cancer itself.

In Cuba, experiments with shark cartilage and late-stage cancer have been going on since 1992, engineered in part by Lane. To date, this work has not been published in medical journals, although Lane's book goes into some detail about the Cuban experiment.[18] Of the original twenty-nine patients, five had late-stage breast cancer. Two of these died of their cancers during the study and another showed new tumor growth; one chose to drop out, but we're not told why. Only one of the five breast cancer patients had a reduction in tumor size. After thirty-five weeks of follow-up, twenty out of the original twenty-nine late-stage Cuban patients were still alive.[19] Lane is hoping to get these results published soon. Only time will tell whether any of these patients will be cured as a result of the cartilage treatment.

Virtually nothing is known yet about the use of shark cartilage to treat early-stage breast cancer. In late-stage disease, the two positive changes that have been anecdotally reported are reduction in tumor size and decreased pain. The former observation may mean little, because endless chemotherapy research has taught us that tumor shrinkage or even short-term disappearance does not mean cure. The latter observation has no immediate meaning for early-stage patients; if you have early-stage breast cancer, you're usually not in pain except for side effects from conventional treatment. Moreover, these studies were done without a placebo control group. Placebo is noted for its ability to "reduce pain."

I have spoken to doctors experimenting with shark cartilage who do not wish to be quoted. The consensus I've heard seems to be that this is no cure-all. Because of all these uncertainties and because a daily dose of 30 to 60 grams of shark cartilage may cost between $15 and $40, I believe that early-stage breast cancer patients should not use this therapy until more is known.

THE GERSON THERAPY

Max Gerson was a European medical doctor who used nutrition successfully to treat his own tuberculosis and reported finding a similar protocol successful with some cancer patients. He fled Nazi Germany and for the rest of his life practiced here in the United States. The Gerson therapy is famous for a very restricted diet, including no salt whatsoever, coffee enemas, and a variety of juices. Although the therapy is used to treat many diseases, it is best known for treating cancer.

In Gerson's book, published in 1958, fifty successful cancer cases were reported, including five breast cancer patients.[20] A subsequent report in 1981, again coming from the Gerson Institute itself, described an additional fifty patients, many of whom did not have cancer and none of whom had cancer of the breast.[21] Neither report indicated how many patients were treated before fifty successful cases could be assembled — a critical issue, as we shall see. An independent assessment of twenty-seven Gerson patients' records was made by English researchers in 1990.[22] The results reported "low pain scores and analgesic requirements" on the one hand, but "little objective evidence of an antitumour effect" on the other. However, all twenty-seven cases came from a group of 149 cases handpicked by the Gerson Institute. Two of the twenty-seven had breast cancer, but neither was considered assessable.

The Gerson therapy anticipated much of what researchers were later to discover about what causes and prevents cancer. Gerson's approach includes abstaining from alcohol, tobacco, red meat, smoked foods, and pickled foods, all of which have now been implicated, even by the ACS, in increased cancer risk. Moreover, the Gerson diet is very high in vitamin A, beta-carotene, vitamin C, fiber, fruits, and vegetables — all of which have more recently been associated with protection against a wide variety of cancers. Most conventional research groups would have to acknowledge such a diet would be useful in *preventing* cancer; I believed it was worthy of investigation as a treatment protocol.

As with the Contreras Hospital, my colleagues and I followed consecutive patients who attended the Gerson clinic in Mexico.[23] We were able to stay in contact with eighteen patients for five years. Seventeen of them died during this time, including all six breast cancer patients. Most alternative doctors believe that the immunosuppressive effects of conventional therapies detract from the therapeutic effects of alternative medicine, so it's interesting to note that though some of these patients had had only limited allopathic (conventional) care, the results were still dismal.

These negative results surprised us. Promising Gerson anecdotes are heard from time to time in alternative medicine circles. In fact, I have met one of the second set of "fifty survivors," and she was in good health. Anecdotes, however, are a very poor way to assess a therapy. The successful former patients survive to tell their tale, but nothing is heard from those who didn't make it. It is often difficult in retrospect to prove that a patient was properly diagnosed and did, in fact, have cancer. Moreover, any therapy will appear to help someone if enough patients are followed. For example, conventional medical treatment for pancreatic cancer is almost always a failure; yet, statistically, if one followed twenty patients with this condition treated by medical doctors, on average, one of them would be alive five years later and therefore appear to be a "success." There is little reason to believe that the patient would have done worse if left untreated.

Even though we followed a very small sample, we observed such consistently poor outcomes that I feel comfortable in steering breast cancer patients away from the Gerson therapy. It remains unknown, from our limited survey, whether the Gerson approach would be of any use to early-stage patients; while fewer of the patients we followed were terminal at the onset of their alternative therapy (in comparison with those at the laetrile clinic), most were late-stage, and none of the breast cancer patients presented with cancer-free nodes.

THE MACROBIOTIC DIET

In the 1960s, the macrobiotic diet became popular in America. It was originally called the "Zen macrobiotic diet," perhaps because American youth were interested in Zen Buddhism at the time. (In fact, the staple food in the macrobiotic program, brown rice, is almost never eaten by real Zen monks in Japan — they eat the same white rice consumed by other Japanese.)

Conventional medicine reacted strongly and swiftly against the macrobiotic approach, which has the distinction of appearing twice on the Questionable Methods list — a testament to its public popularity.[24,25] In a position paper against the diet, the American Medical Association (AMA) has called it "one of the most dangerous dietary regimens, posing not only serious hazards to the health of the individual but even to life itself."[26]

The diet *can* be deficient in vitamin B_{12},[27] calcium, and vitamin D.[28] Yet almost all components of the typical American diet that have been linked to cancer and other chronic diseases are excluded from the macrobiotic approach. This fact was never mentioned in AMA or ACS attacks. The AMA position paper is almost embarrassing in the transparency of its conflict of interest. It tells us "the greatest danger for followers of the Zen macrobiotics philosophy [is that] medical consultation is not advocated." In cynical moments, I've wondered if perhaps the AMA does not similarly condemn junk food, red meat, and dairy fat because they have the opposite effect — to bring in more business.

What is the macrobiotic approach, and why is conventional medicine so reactive to it? The diet, based loosely on the old oriental philosophy of opposites (yin and yang), contains much brown rice, lots of vegetables (including sea vegetation), soy products (including salty miso and soy sauce), a little fish, and not much else.

Some of its tenets are clearly off-base. For example, fruit is discouraged, and orange juice is considered cancer-causing. The relationship between fruit (including citrus) and cancer has been extensively studied by researchers, and it is clear that fruit protects against many cancers.[29] Macrobiotic proponents have been quite mild in their condemnation of smoking. Yet rarely has any health issue been so well-studied or found to be so directly linked to serious diseases.

The current leader of the macrobiotic movement, Michio Kushi, has said that cancer can be caused by "eating too much fish" and that lung cancer is linked to "fat and mucus."[30] In other words, macrobiotic proponents don't even pay lip service to scientific reality.

Like the Gerson diet, however, macrobiotics eliminates red meat, dairy fat, alcohol, low-fiber foods, high-fat foods, and many other dietary components linked with cancer. Also like the Gerson regimen, it is high in protective antioxidants (see Chapter 13). Therefore, it has piqued the interest of alternative practitioners as a possible cancer therapy, and reports of successfully treated cases have appeared in the alternative medical press.[31]

One recent report studied survival in patients with prostate and pancreatic cancers who ate a macrobiotic diet.[32] These cases were compared with a control group compiled from SEER (Surveillance Epidemiology and End Results) National Tumor Registry statistics. Although most late-stage patients on the macrobiotic program eventually died, the macrobiotic group clearly outlived the control group. Average survival in twenty-three pancreatic cancer patients was seventeen months compared with six months for the SEER controls. The eighteen prostate cancer patients lived an average of 177 months compared with 91 months in the control group.

These patients were not randomly chosen to use the macrobiotic diet, and therefore it can be argued they may not have
been representative of other cancer patients. Almost nothing is
known about macrobiotics and breast cancer specifically.
Nonetheless, the results suggest that this dietary approach should
at least be studied further.

In Chapter 12, I'll review the research showing how diet is
linked with breast cancer and suggest dietary changes to reduce
the risk of a recurrence. Many of these changes will mimic aspects of the low-fat, high-fiber macrobiotic program. Wherever
science diverges from the macrobiotic approach, however, I
choose to go with the science. Why not enjoy fruit when it is
good for your overall health and is associated with a lower cancer
risk?

THE HOXSEY FORMULA

Another well-known alternative therapy, the Hoxsey treatment,
uses primarily herbs. Harry Hoxsey called himself a naturopathic
doctor, though he was an unlicensed practitioner with a dubious
diploma. Hoxsey used an old veterinary anticancer herbal formula passed down in his family. He was the first to treat humans
with these plant extracts. As a result of pressure from the AMA, he
was repeatedly charged with practicing medicine without a li-
cense. In all probability, the charges were technically valid, but
he was never convicted. Hoxsey's lawyers would parade successfully treated patients in front of the juries and so convince them
to vote "not guilty."

Much of the treatment (and courtroom saga) was described
for lay people in Hoxsey's book, *You Don't Have to Die.*[33] Some of
the herbs, such as licorice root, poke root, and barberry, have
subsequently been found to contain anticancer or immune-stimu-
lating substances.[34-37] Others, like red clover, were used to treat
cancer in traditional Native American medicine. The reason for including some of the other constituents, however, remains somewhat of a mystery, because the formula (at least for veterinary
use) goes back 150 years. Harry Hoxsey, the great-grandson of

the formulator, has been considered the quintessential quack by the AMA, and the therapy remains on the Questionable Methods list. Frankly, the sensational tone of Hoxsey's book doesn't engender confidence. Nonetheless, although the ACS claims that the Hoxsey formula has been "extensively tested" and found "useless,"[38] it cites no scientific studies to support its claim — resorting, rather, to the transcripts of several old court cases, which by no stretch of the imagination constitute "extensive" testing.

In our 1983–88 study, my colleagues and I were able to follow sixteen cancer patients at the Biomedical Center in Tijuana, Mexico, where the Hoxsey treatment is now used.[39] All had had cancer diagnosed through biopsy in the United States before treatment began. After a follow-up that averaged fifty-eight months, ten had died of cancer. Two of the six surviving patients clearly had had fatal prognoses (advanced lung cancer and level V melanoma); the other four had had skin cancer, a recurrent bladder cancer, melanoma, and lung cancer for which we had little staging information. None of the six had had breast cancer. All six (by written survey) believed themselves to be cancer-free at 48 to 96 months after starting the Hoxsey treatment. Even if their self-assessments are incorrect, their mere survival is a surprise.

We used no control group when making our preliminary observation. But the result is unlikely to be due to placebo effect alone. Long-term survival for patients diagnosed with advanced lung cancer and level V melanoma is rare indeed.

Taken by themselves, these cases should be interesting enough to elicit attention from researchers concerned with finding viable cancer therapies. But the medical community has notorious disregard for botanical (herbal) medicine, despite the fact that many modern prescription medicines are derived from or modeled after substances in plants. It is particularly paradoxical that oncologists spurn herbal products when conventional anti-cancer drugs like vincristine and taxol are themselves herbal extracts. Nevertheless, the bias of conventional medicine against botanicals, like disdain for Hoxsey himself, probably precludes the possibility that the Hoxsey formula will be seriously investigated in the near future.

What about Hoxsey and breast cancer? Two patients were not included in our final results because their "breast cancers" had never been biopsied. Despite the fact that both had signs suggesting cancer but remained clinically well, these anecdotes weren't counted. One of the ten who eventually died (of colon cancer) reported that she had been successfully treated by Hoxsey for breast cancer fourteen years earlier; her anecdote is also not considered in the numbers presented above. One of the ten who died had had late-stage breast cancer when she began the Hoxsey treatment. While we believe these results warrant further investigation, there aren't enough data here to form any definitive conclusions.

If you're wondering whether Cathy takes the herbs listed in Hoxsey's book, she does. Finding between two and six miracles in a group of 16 cancer patients has impressed us, though none of the six had breast cancer. Although the results of our study look promising, they are very far from conclusive and it would be unwise to read the Hoxsey book and take the herbs on your own. Iodine is included with the herbal preparation, and it can be toxic, as can one of the herbal constituents, phytolacca.

If you have an interest, I suggest you start by discussing it with a licensed naturopathic physician. A call to one of the accredited four-year naturopathic colleges — Bastyr College in Seattle (206-523-9585), National College of Naturopathic Medicine in Portland, Oregon (503-255-4860), the new Southwest College of Naturopathic Medicine in Scottsdale, Arizona (602-990-7424), or to the Canadian College of Naturopathic Medicine in Etobicoke, Ontario (416-251-5261) — or the American Association of Naturopathic Physicians in Seattle (206-323-7610) would be helpful in establishing a local lead.

It's also possible to receive the Hoxsey treatment in Tijuana. I'm hesitant to suggest that early-stage breast cancer patients consider making the trip. While the initial clinic visit may take only a day or two, the cost of the whole treatment is considerable (several thousand dollars), and repeated trips to Mexico may be necessary. Also, to my knowledge, the herbs used at the Biomedical Center in Tijuana are no different from those on the list reported in Hoxsey's book; in other words, doctors well-versed in the use of herbs should be able to produce a facsimile of the formula by reading Hoxsey's book. (In fact, several formulas are commercially available.) Moreover, for early-stage breast cancer, unlike topical (skin) cancers, the only special treatment used at the Biomedical Center is the herbal formula.

Though the Biomedical Center in Tijuana does suggest a diet, it was not part of the original Hoxsey treatment, nor does it fit with what we currently know about cancer and nutrition. A few supplements are also included, but at least one of them, iron, may actually be counterproductive (see Chapter 13).

Occasionally, a medical anecdote is worth repeating. I found it interesting that almost every patient I interviewed at the Biomedical Center claimed to personally know someone who had had cancer diagnosed in the States and had then been successfully treated with the Hoxsey approach. At the other clinics we visited, such word-of-mouth advertisement was much rarer; patients had come to the clinics because of something they had read or heard in a lecture.

Hoxsey always claimed that his treatment worked best for topical (skin) cancers, including melanoma. Although we might speculate that this success occurs because many topical cancers are not life-threatening, melanoma frequently is. In our small sample, two of three melanoma patients reported long-term disease-free survival, and one of them had level V (advanced) disease at the start of the therapy. Although this proves nothing, it suggests to me that studying the Hoxsey formula makes more sense than deriding it.

LINUS PAULING AND VITAMIN C THERAPY

Several vitamins and minerals called antioxidants protect the body against a form of cellular damage linked with cancer. As we see in Chapter 13, each of these vitamin and mineral antioxidants, including vitamin C, appears to provide some protection against cancer. Vitamin C is also known to protect animals from cancer.[40,41,42] It is now relatively well accepted that vitamin C protects humans from stomach cancer.[43,44,45] Many researchers believe other cancer risks are also reduced by higher-than-normal vitamin C intake.[46]

Vitamin C affects the immune system, which must be functioning well to combat cancer. White blood cells (WBCs), the immune system's primary fighting force, contain the vitamin. Reviews of the research show that WBCs taken from cancer patients have less vitamin C than do WBCs from healthy people.[47,48]

Treating cancer with vitamin C has been a controversial issue since Linus Pauling, the Nobel Prize-winning scientist, began to advocate it years ago. Working with a Scottish surgeon, Ewan Cameron, Pauling decided to investigate the possibility that vitamin C might help patients who already have cancer.[49] One hundred terminal cancer patients were given 10 grams of vitamin C daily (2.5 grams four times per day) and followed until death. They lived an average of 210 days, compared with hospital records of 1,000 "matched controls" (similar patients) who averaged only 50 days. A follow-up showed an even wider gap between the vitamin C and control groups.[50]

The rest of the research community was concerned about these results, in part because the 1,000 control patients received no placebo.[51] In other words, the patients taking the vitamin might have lived longer because they believed the therapy might have helped them.* Ironically, while conventional medicine has very little interest in psychological intervention in cancer treatment, medical doctors feel no qualms about using the argument that placebo effect, a psychological intervention, might extend life significantly.

_____

*In a placebo-controlled trial, all patients know they might be receiving a treatment or they might be getting an inert placebo. The function of such a control is to remove the psychological advantage of getting *something* from the purely physical effects of the treatment. Because patients don't know whether they've received the real treatment or the placebo, the real treatment group has no psychological advantage over the placebo group. Otherwise there would be a bias; it is well known that people who merely think they have received a real treatment often do better physically.

The Mayo Clinic attempted to test Cameron and Pauling's results. The Mayo Clinic paper, which did have a placebo-control group, reported that vitamin C did not help.[52] Linus Pauling protested that the two trials weren't equivalent because most of the Mayo Clinic patients had had chemotherapy, while his patients had not. This distinction might be important because chemotherapy impairs the immune system; and, as mentioned earlier, one way in which vitamin C might help cancer patients is by boosting immune function. Theoretically, a damaged immune system might not be able to take advantage of supplemental vitamin C.

In response, the Mayo Clinic proceeded to do another study testing vitamin C. This time they used patients who had had no chemotherapy.[53] The researchers said that this trial was ethical because "there is no known form of chemotherapy for colorectal cancer that has been demonstrated to produce substantive palliative benefit or extension of survival."[54] For this reason, the second Mayo Clinic study was limited to colon cancer patients. Once again, the researchers claimed that vitamin C was useless.

But careful examination of the second Mayo clinic study shows that Pauling's hypothesis was never tested. Pauling said that terminal cancer patients fed vitamin C until death would live substantially longer. In the Mayo study, as soon as the cancer progressed, patients were taken off vitamin C. The researchers claimed that it was unethical to keep them on the therapy because it wasn't working. In fact, there was no way to know whether the vitamin C was "working" unless patients were kept on it until they died. Keep in mind that these were terminal patients to begin with. Pauling and Cameron had never said that the vitamin was curative (though a couple of their patients actually lived for many years); rather, they claimed only that terminal patients taking C until they died lived longer on average.

There was another irony in the stance taken by the Mayo Clinic team. While it was "inhumane" to keep patients on vitamin C,[55] an inexpensive and harmless supplement, many of these patients were subsequently given fluorouracil, the very form of chemotherapy that had been proven repeatedly to be ineffectual

and toxic in the treatment of colon cancer. Recall that the uselessness of chemo was the initial ethical justification for putting terminal colon cancer patients on a regimen that did not include
chemo. Although the transparency of the clinic researchers' bias
has been discussed in relatively obscure alternative sources,[56] it
has not been picked up by the media or by conventional medical
journals.

A separate criticism of the second Mayo Clinic trial also has
some merit: The control group may also have been taking vitamin
C. All of the colon cancer patients were told that vitamin C was
being tested to see if it would help them. They were also told that
they might not be getting the real vitamin C; their pill might be
just a placebo. Under these circumstances, who would be so
compliant as to not sneak a little vitamin C on the side? Such a
surreptitious change would obviously invalidate the outcome. A
very limited investigation was made to rule out this possibility
(only six placebo-taking patients were checked, and they were
checked at only one point in time). Vitamin C excreted in urine
reflects oral intake; patients were considered not to be taking
clandestine vitamin C if their urine contained 550 milligrams of vitamin C per day or less — vastly more than the average person
will excrete under normal circumstances. It seems inconceivable
that the Mayo researchers didn't know that fact. Even at the 550
milligram level, one of the six patients exceeded the limit,
strongly suggesting that he or she was "cheating," as most thinking people would do under the circumstances. To restate the implications, patients in the placebo group could have been taking
vitamin C; and the test the researchers used to rule that out was
faulty.

The Mayo Clinic's bias is revealed in other ways as well. In
their *New England Journal* report, the researchers state, "It is very
clear that this study fails to show a benefit for high-dose vitamin
C therapy of advanced cancer."[57] The study doesn't deal with "advanced cancer" as stated — only with colon cancer. This might
seem to be a minor detail, but it's the very kind of technicality
that researchers are extremely careful of in order to protect themselves from future criticism. It's uncommon for researchers to

overstate their case in the *New England Journal of Medicine;* it seems plausible that this exaggeration was included to affect the press more than to inform scientists and doctors.

Normally, scientists work together in an environment of collegiality. Typically, those working in the same field are in close touch and usually know how colleagues' efforts are proceeding even before work is published. To purposely keep a scientist of the caliber of Linus Pauling in the dark is both unusual and very poor form, to say the least; yet this is apparently what the Mayo Clinic did. In a press release, Pauling

> expressed his concern about the behaviour of the Mayo Clinic physicians in taking positive steps to prevent him and Dr. Cameron from learning about the nature of the Mayo Clinic work until it had been published. The principal investigator in the Mayo Clinic work had promised Dr. Pauling that he would provide a copy of the paper to Dr. Pauling and Dr. Cameron before the date of publication, but then he did not do so.[58]

Frequently unmentioned in the ongoing debate between Linus Pauling and the Mayo Clinic is the fact that Pauling's work has already been independently verified by Japanese researchers. Murata and Morishige's high doses of vitamin C (five grams or more per day) extended patients' lives from an average of 43 to 246 days,[59] a change remarkably similar to that reported by Cameron and Pauling.

While the issue has not been resolved (the Japanese study also lacked a placebo control), the characterization that "vitamin C goes down for the count" that appeared in the medical press[60] is more wish than fact.

If we focus on what effect vitamin C had on breast cancer patients in the Pauling study, we find survival times of more than 487 days versus 52 days.[61] Keep in mind that these patients were terminal. These figures tell us very little about using vitamin C to treat early-stage disease. Although we may speculate that a substance that extends life in late-stage cancer patients might do better at an earlier point in time, especially because there is much evidence that vitamin C prevents cancer,[62] we have no facts to back up this assumption. A study exploring this possibility would take years and require considerable funding — money that's currently unavailable for this kind of research.

As you might expect, Cathy takes 12 grams of vitamin C every day "just in case." The only common side effect, diarrhea, can be controlled by simply lowering the dose. Possible links between large doses of vitamin C and kidney stones have been suggested; but in the absence of a history of such stones, vitamin C appears to be relatively safe. Avoid the chewable form of vitamin C. It usually contains sugar, and the combination of the acid in the vitamin and the added sugar can cause tooth decay. If you're considering taking vitamin C and have had problems with diarrhea or a history of kidney stones, it's particularly important to talk with a nutrition-oriented doctor. Graduates of some chiropractic colleges (such as Western States or Los Angeles Chiropractic College) or any licensed naturopathic physician should be well-versed in vitamin C supplementation.

PSYCHOLOGICAL INTERVENTION

Much has been written about whether a "cancer personality" exists. The ACS-published review of this material downplays the possible link between cancer and personality,[63] though other reviewers seem to be finding such a connection.[64,65] The issue has yet to be resolved.[66] In any case, several research groups report that the basic personality of a breast cancer patient does not affect her survival.[67,68,69] The question should not be, Do you have the cancer personality? or, in the more sinister version, Did you "cause" your cancer? Rather, the important issue is this: Does involving the mind in the treatment process through counseling, guided imagery, or any other nonphysical intervention extend life and/or improve its quality?

In 1989, the *Lancet* published research exploring the effects of psychological intervention in treating late-stage breast cancer.[70] For one year, fifty such patients were placed in a professionally led support group that met for ninety minutes once a week. Statistically, all of these patients should have died. Even though the group was disbanded at the end of the year and surviving patients were left to fend for themselves, three were still alive ten years later, and the average length of survival among the fifty was twice as long as thirty-six matched breast cancer patients who were not psychologically supported at all. All thirty-six women in the control group died as expected.

Statistically, the difference was highly significant. Interestingly, the study was apparently undertaken for the purpose of showing that the mind was not likely to affect the body! When the chief author was asked to explain what happened, the journal *Science* paraphrased his response: "The therapy may have caused a change in mental attitude that made the subjects comply better with their doctors' orders regarding medication and diet."[71] The reaction from the chief psychiatrist at Memorial Sloan-Kettering Cancer Center was, "what I am fearful of is that the 'alternative' field will go crazy with this."[72]

Apparently, hardly anyone was initially pleased by the fact that life expectancy doubled — a feat unmatched by any conventional treatments of late-stage breast cancer. It should be noted, however, that the principal investigator, David Spiegel, has now become somewhat more of an advocate for psychological intervention.

How does the mind affect the body? If you've ever noticed that you're more likely to catch a cold when stressed out, you understand that the mind influences immunity. An entire new field of research called psychoneuroimmunology is exploring these links. The immune system can protect us from cancer. Stress reduces natural killer cell activity — one expression of the body's ability to mount an immune response against cancer cells. Researchers at the University of Pittsburgh School of Medicine have found that natural killer cell activity is also reduced by depression and lack of social support.[73] Those patients who feel that they're getting good support from spouses and doctors have stronger immune systems as a result, as demonstrated by statistically higher levels of activity by natural killer cells.[74]

Researchers have shown that some breast cancer patients who experience a severely stressful event after their diagnosis (such as the death of a spouse or child, divorce, etc.) are more likely to have a recurrence,[75,76] though inconsistencies exist in some studies[77] and a recent study found no correlation whatever.[78]

English researcher Steven Greer and his coworkers, in a series of articles, have shown that *the way a patient chooses to psychologically respond to her breast cancer diagnosis determines the outcome more than any other single factor, including initial staging.*[79,80] In this fifteen-year study, patients with a fighting attitude had the best chance of survival. Those in denial also did well. Stoic acceptance was associated with a lower chance of survival, and a helpless/hopeless attitude was accompanied by the worst chance of survival. The attitudes of stoicism and helpless/hopelessness were not associated with a more advanced stage or worse medical prognosis; in other words, there is reason to believe that the attitude affected the outcome rather than that the expected outcome affected the attitude.[81] At the end of fifteen years, patients who chose to fight or deny had more than two and a half times the chance of being alive that stoics and those without hope had.[82] Furthermore, these researchers have recently shown that the attitude of cancer patients can be improved through psychological intervention;[83] in other words, you aren't stuck with a poor attitude just because it's habitual. The improvement included more "fighting spirit" — the very attitude associated with the longest survival!

By focusing on modifying breast cancer patients' reactions to stress, Grossarth-Maticek and Eysenck, European researchers, have also increased survival times for late-stage patients. This study reported that immune function increased in those patients receiving the psychological intervention.[84] Other researchers have also reported that psychological intervention improves immune function in cancer patients.[85]

An additional study has indirectly confirmed that fighters (as defined by "increased hostility" and "poorer attitudes" toward their physicians) live longer.[86] And there is also evidence that psychological intervention helps patients feel better physically.[87]

If by now, you're interested in psychological intervention, what can you do? Don't worry about your past. Remember, it has been shown that your prior personality doesn't seem to affect your survival. The issue is how you cope with your diagnosis and what psychological tools you use in helping yourself. Several methods are available.

The most famous is the Simonton approach. In their book, *Getting Well Again,* O. Carl Simonton, a medical doctor, and Stephanie Mathews-Simonton, a counselor, advocate combining psychological intervention with conventional medical methods.[88] Among other approaches, they use guided imagery — a way to visualize one's immune system defeating the cancer. The Simonton book includes sections on relaxation, overcoming resentment, and looking forward by setting future goals. If you're interested in the Simonton method, the first step is to read the book. Be forewarned that a minority of readers respond with a sense of guilt — they feel the tie between attitude and cancer means they "caused" their disease. If you're engulfed by such a response, perhaps another approach is in order, even if the methods appeal to you.

The Simonton Cancer Center in Pacific Palisades, California (310-459-4434) can provide you with the name of a professional counselor in your area who has been specially trained by Carl Simonton to work with cancer patients using this approach. Stephanie Simonton, at the Behavioral Medicine Program in Little Rock, Arkansas (501-686-8700), will also provide local referrals. Guided imagery tapes associated with Carl's work are available from a toll-free number (800-338-2360). Tapes put together by Stephanie can be obtained by calling the Arkansas number.

It has been our experience that Simonton-trained counselors are very helpful in working out psychological approaches to treatment. Interestingly, the Simontons have published data showing results from their intervention similar to those achieved by the support group approach mentioned earlier:[89] a doubling of life expectancy in late-stage breast cancer.[90] It seems remarkable that while this statistic beats any conventional therapies, the medical community is still hostile toward considering the effects of psychological intervention.

Another popular book in the field, also written by a medical doctor, is Bernie Siegel's *Love, Medicine, and Miracles.*[91] Siegel's book is less structured and more narrative than the Simontons'. Some patients are more comfortable with one over the other; but, in our experience, most people get something useful from both. As with the reactions to Simonton, a few readers of Siegel's book respond primarily with a sense of responsibility or guilt, though in neither case is this the intention of the authors. Understand-ably, the line between what is said (your mind can affect your body) and what is sometimes heard (you caused your disease) can become fuzzy for some people caught in the emotional storm of a cancer diagnosis. Nonetheless, we strongly recommend read-ing *Love, Medicine, and Miracles.*

In some cities, ECaP (exceptional cancer patients) groups have evolved from Siegel's book. Sometimes the social workers at local hospitals can steer you toward an ECaP group.

As you might guess, Cathy uses psychological intervention in her treatment. Initially, she went into therapy to work on the fears and stresses resulting from the diagnosis; later, she attended an ECaP-like group. For years, she used both relaxation and guided imagery tapes on a daily basis, and now she meditates instead. And, as a counselor, she works with cancer patients herself.

Before leaving psychological intervention, I'd like to point out that all seven of the articles I cited that show therapeutic ef-fects from psychological intervention were published outside the United States.[92-98] This may not be coincidental. It's my experience that medical journals coming from countries other than the United States or Canada typically have a more open-minded editorial policy and are consequently more willing to consider a variety of alternative approaches.

OTHER ALTERNATIVE THERAPIES

In 1975, Eydie Mae, a breast cancer patient, wrote a book — *How I Conquered Cancer Naturally* — about her survival after at-tending the Hippocrates Institute in Boston.[99] The treatment in-cludes the use of wheatgrass juice and a diet that excludes meat, alcohol, caffeine, etc. Unlike the Gerson therapy, emphasis is placed on the difference between raw ("good") and cooked ("bad") food. Conventional research has not looked at this distinction in relation to cancer. Moreover, when we attempted to follow attendees at the Health Institute of San Diego (which is similar to the Hippocrates Institute), we were not permitted to do so. Therefore, it's impossible for me to evaluate this approach.

American Biologics Hospital uses a variety of therapies, centered on a variation of the metabolic approach that proved so unsuccessful at the Contreras Hospital. American Biologics also did not permit us to follow patients.

At the Harold Manner Clinic, there weren't enough appropriate patients for us to study during our short stay. As a result, we have no useful information. Because the Manner Clinic also uses a variation on the metabolic therapy, however, it would seem prudent, based on our experience, to avoid it.

The Livingston-Wheeler Clinic in San Diego views cancer as an infection and uses a treatment based on increasing immunological function. As with the Manner Clinic, at the time of our visit there were not enough patients for us to meaningfully evaluate. A recent study of late-stage cancer patients who attended the Livingston-Wheeler Clinic indicates that they did just as poorly as if they had continued to be treated by conventional medical doctors.[100]

Many other alternative treatments exist, such as the work done at the clinics of Emmanuel Revici in New York and Hans Nieper in Germany. While I have heard impressive anecdotes about the Revici clinic, I have no specific information. To my knowledge, no patients have been studied independently in any in-depth fashion. I suggest that you be leery of miracle stories when you have nothing else to go on and no real sense of what percentage of breast cancer patients do well.

Recent books on alternative therapies may provide more information.[101,102] However, in considering the evaluations of these therapies, it is critical to remember that prevention is not the same as treatment, and research with rat liver enzymes done in a test tube is not the same as human research.

To review, conventional medical research groups have avoided evaluating alternatives. Small, independent inquiries directed at filling in the blanks have shown the results of several specific alternative therapies to be less than promising. Sound discouraging? Not necessarily for early-stage patients, who will often be disease-free after whatever conventional treatment is chosen. For such patients, the issue may not be looking for a way to treat cancer with alternatives, but rather for a way to prevent a recurrence. Although it's rare for a surgeon or oncologist to mention any of the many ways in which you might possibly reduce your risk of a recurrence, much encouraging research exists and will be detailed in subsequent chapters.

And for all breast cancer patients, regardless of stage, psychological intervention can be of enormous importance.

References

1. Chowka, P., et al. The NIH's new office of alternative medicine: hope or hype? American Association of Naturopathic Physicians' Annual Convention, September 4, 1993, Portland, Oregon.
2. Epstein, S. S. *The politics of cancer.* Anchor Press/Doubleday, Garden City, NY, 1979.
3. Moertel, C. G., et al. A clinical trial of amygdalin (Laetrile) in the treatment of human cancer. *N Engl J Med* 1982;306:201–6.
4. Rorvik, D. The politics of cancer: laetrile — the drug that never was. *Penthouse* January 1981.
5. Manner, H. W. Tumor regression with laetrile therapy. *J Internat Acad Prevent Med* Winter, 1983:48–50.
6. Austin, S., E. Baumgartner Dale, and S. DeKadt. Long term follow-up of cancer patients from Contreras, Gerson and Hoxsey clinics. *J Naturopathic Med,* in press.
7. Austin, S. Negative long-term outcome in nine of ten patients using combined laetrile/metabolic approach. *Townsend Letter for Doctors* 1984; #17:146 [letter].
8. Austin, S., E. Baumgartner, and S. DeKadt. Monitoring of cancer patients treated with laetrile. *Townsend Letter for Doctors* 1991;#101:1005 [letter].
9. Prudden, J. F. The treatment of human cancer with agents prepared from bovine cartilage. *J Biol Response Modifiers* 1985;4:551–84.
10. Lane, I. W., and L. Comac. *Sharks don't get cancer.* Avery Publishing, Garden City Park, NY, 1993.
11. Lee, A., and R. Langer. Shark cartilage contains inhibitors of tumor angiogenesis. *Science* 1983;221:1185–7.

12. Moses, M. A., J. Sudhalter, and R. Langer. Identification of an inhibitor of neovascularization from cartilage. *Science* 1990;248:1408–10.

13. Lane, I. W. Shark cartilage: its potential medical applications. *J Advancement in Med* 1991;4:263–271.

14. Lane, I. W., and E. Contreras, Jr. High rate of bioactivity (reduction in gross tumor size) observed in advanced cancer patients treated with shark cartilage material. *J Naturopathic Med* 1992;3:86–8.

15. Lane, I. W. Personal communication.

16. Lane, I. W., and L. Comac. *Sharks don't get cancer.* Avery Publishing, Garden City Park, NY, 1993, p. 99.

17. Van Zandt, R. L. Personal communication.

18. Lane, I. W., and L. Comac. *Sharks don't get cancer.* Avery Publishing, Garden City Park, NY, 1993, pp. 101–107.

19. Lane, I. W. Personal communications.

20. Gerson, M. *A cancer therapy — results of fifty cases.* Third Edition. Totality Books, Del Mar, CA, 1977.

21. Fifty healed "incurables." *Healing* 1981;1(1):3,4,6,9,13–22.

22. Reed, A., et al. Mexico: juices, coffee enemas, and cancer. *Lancet* 1990; 336:677–8.

23. Austin, S., E. Baumgartner Dale, and S. DeKadt. Long term follow-up of cancer patients from Contreras, Gerson and Hoxsey clinics. *J Naturopathic Med,* in press.

24. Unproven methods of cancer management: macrobiotic diets. *CA* 1984; 34:60–3.

25. Unproven methods of cancer management: macrobiotic diets for the treatment of cancer. *CA* 1989;39:248–51.

26. AMA Council on Foods and Nutrition. Zen macrobiotic diets. *JAMA* 1971;218:397.

27. Miller, D. R., et al. Vitamin B-12 status in a macrobiotic community. *Am J Clin Nutr* 1991;53:524–9.

28. Dwyer, J. T., et al. Risk of nutritional rickets among vegetarian children. *Am J Dis Child* 1979;133:134–40.

29. Block, G., B. Patterson, and A. Subar. Fruit, vegetables, and cancer prevention: a review of the epidemiological evidence. *Nutr Cancer* 1992; 18:1–29.

30. The challenge of cancer. *East West J* March,1983; pp. 34–44.

31. Newbold, V. Complete remission of advanced medically incurable cancer in six patients following a macrobiotic approach to healing. *Townsend Letter for Doctors.* October, 1990; pp. 638–43.

32. Carter, J. P., et al. Hypothesis: dietary management may improve survival

from nutritionally linked cancers based on analysis of representative cases. *J Am Coll Nutr* 1993;12:209–26.

33. Hoxsey, H. *You don't have to die.* Milestone Books, New York, 1956.

34. Kitagawa, K., et al. Inhibition of the specific binding of 12-0-tetrade-canoylphorbol-13-acetate to mouse epidermal membrane fractions by glycerrhetic acid. *Oncology* 1986;43:127–30.

35. Nishino, H., et al. Antitumor activity of glycerrhetic acid in mouse skin tumor promotion induces 7,12-demethylbenz[a]anthracene plus teleocidin. *Carcinogenesis* 1984;5:1529–30.

36. Hoshi, A., et al. Antitumor activity of berberine derivatives. *Japan J Cancer Res* 1976;67:321–5.

37. Zhang, J. P., Qian D-H, Zheng Q-Y. Effects of phytolacca acinosa polysaccharides I on cytotoxicity of macrophages and its production of tumor necrosis factor and interleukin 1. *Acta Pharmacologica Sinica* 1990;11:375–7.

38. Hoxsey method/bio-medical center. *CA* 1990;40(1):51–55.

39. Austin, S., E. Baumgartner Dale, and S. DeKadt. Long term follow-up of cancer patients from Contreras, Gerson and Hoxsey Clinics. *J Naturopathic Med,* in press.

40. Pavelic, K. L-ascorbic acid-induced DNA strand breaks and cross links in human neuroblastoma cells. *Brain Res* 1985;342:369–73.

41. Morrison, D. G., et al. Retinyl palmitate and ascorbic acid inhibit pulmonary neoplasms in mice exposed to fiberglass dust. *Nutr Cancer* 1982;3(2):81.

42. Abdel-Galili, A. M. Preventive effect of vitamin C (L-ascorbic acid) on methylcholanthrene-induced soft tissue sarcomas in mice. *Oncology* 1986;43:335–7.

43. Weisburger, J. H. Vitamin C, vitamin E, and the prevention of gastric cancer: discussion. *Ann NY Acad Sci* 1980;355:278–9.

44. Tannenbaum, W., and W. Mergens. Reaction of nitrite with vitamins C and E. *Ann NY Acad Sci* 1980;355:267–75.

45. Weisburger, J. H. Causes of gastric and esophageal cancer. Possible approaches to prevention by vitamin C. *Int J Vit Nutr Res* 1985; Suppl #27:381–402.

46. Block, G. Vitamin C and cancer prevention: the epidemiologic evidence. *Am J Clin Nutr* 1991;53:270S–82S [review].

47. Basu, T. K. The significance of ascorbic acid, thiamin and retinol in cancer. *Int J Vit Nutr Res* 1983; Suppl #24:105–17.

48. Hanck, A. Vitamin C and cancer. *Int J Vit Nutr Res* 1983; Suppl #24:87–104.

49. Cameron, E., and L. Pauling. Supplemental ascorbate in the supportive

treatment of cancer: prolongation of survival times in terminal human cancer. *Proc Natl Acad Sci USA* 1976;73:3685–9.

50. Cameron, E., and L. Pauling. Supplemental ascorbate in the supportive treatment of cancer: reevaluation of prolongation of survival times in terminal human cancer. *Proc Natl Acad Sci USA* 1978;75:4538–42.

51. Moertel, C. G. A proposition: megadoses of vitamin C are valuable in the treatment of cancer — negative. *Nutr Rev* 1986;44(1):29–30.

52. Creagan, E. T., et al. Failure of high dose vitamin C (ascorbic acid) therapy to benefit patients with advanced cancer. *N Engl J Med* 1979;301:687–90.

53. Moertel, C. G., et al. High-dose vitamin C versus placebo in the treatment of patients with advanced cancer who have had no prior chemotherapy: a randomized double-blind comparison. *New Engl J Med* 1985;312(3):137–41.

54. Moertel, C. G., et al. High-dose vitamin C versus placebo in the treatment of patients with advanced cancer who have had no prior chemotherapy: a randomized double-blind comparison. *New Engl J Med* 1985;312(3):137–41.

55. The effects of high dose vitamin C on survival of cancer patients. *Int Clin Nutr Rev* 1985;5(4):163–5 [editorial].

56. Chaitow, L. Vitamin C study on cancer patients "seriously flawed." *J Alternative Med* April 1985, pp. 18–19.

57. Moertel, C. G., et al. High-dose vitamin C versus placebo in the treatment of patients with advanced cancer who have had no prior chemotherapy: a randomized double-blind comparison. *N Engl J Med* 1985;312(3):137–41.

58. The effects of high dose vitamin C on survival of cancer patients. *Int Clin Nutr Rev* 1985;5(4):163–5 [editorial].

59. Murata, A., F. Morishige, and H. Yamaguchi. Prolongation of survival times of terminal cancer patients by administration of large doses of ascorbate. *Int J Vit Nutr Res* 1982; Suppl #23:103–114.

60. Vitamin C goes down for the count in advanced-cancer controlled trial. *Med World News* Aug 22, 1983, p. 69.

61. Cameron, E., and L. Pauling. Ascorbic acid as a therapeutic agent in cancer. *J Internat Acad Prev Med* 1978;5(1):8–29.

62. Block, G. Vitamin C and cancer prevention: the epidemiologic evidence. *Am J Clin Nutr* 1991;53:270S–82S [review].

63. Wellisch, D. K., and J. Yager. Is there a cancer-prone personality? *CA* 1983; 33:145–53.

64. Levy, S. M. Emotions and the progression of cancer: a review. *Advances* 1984;1(1):10–15.

65. Bower, B. The character of cancer. *Sci News* 1987;131:120–121.

66. Jensen, A. B. Psychosocial factors in breast cancer and their possible impact upon prognosis. *Cancer Treat Rev* 1991;18:191–210.

67. Spiegel, D., et al. Effects of psychosocial treatment on survival of patients with metastatic breast cancer. *Lancet* 1989;ii:888–91.
68. Jamison, R. N., et al. Psychogenic factors in predicting survival of breast cancer patients. *J Clin Oncol* 1987;5:768–72.
69. Cassileth, B. R., et al. Psychosocial correlates of survival in advanced malignant disease? *N Engl J Med* 1985;312:1551–5.
70. Spiegel, D., et al. Effects of psychosocial treatment on survival of patients with metastatic breast cancer. *Lancet* 1989;ii:888–91.
71. Barinaga, M. Can psychotherapy delay cancer deaths? *Science* 1989; 246:448–9.
72. Barinaga, M. Can psychotherapy delay cancer deaths? *Science* 1989; 246:448–9.
73. Levy, S., et al. Correlation of stress factors with sustained depression of natural killer cell activity and predicted prognosis in patients with breast cancer. *J Clin Oncol* 1987;5:348–53.
74. Levy, S., et al. Perceived social support and tumor estrogen/progesterone receptor status as predictors of natural killer cell activity in breast cancer patients. *Psychosomatic Med* 1990;52:73–85.
75. Ramirez, A. J., et al. Stress and relapse of breast cancer. *BMJ* 1989; 298:291–3.
76. Ramirez, A. J., et al. Psychological correlates of hormone receptor status in breast cancer. *Lancet* 1990;335:1408 [letter].
77. Jensen, A. B. Psychosocial factors in breast cancer and their possible impact upon prognosis. *Cancer Treat Rev* 1991;18:191–210.
78. Barraclough, J., et al. Life events and breast cancer prognosis. *BMJ* 1993;307:325 [letter].
79. Greer, S., et al. Psychological response to breast cancer: effect on outcome. *Lancet* 1979;ii:785–7.
80. Greer, S., et al. Psychological response to breast cancer and 15-year outcome. *Lancet* 1990;335:49–50 [letter].
81. Pettingale, K. W., et al. Psychological response to cancer diagnosis — I. correlations with prognostic variables. *J Psychosomatic Res* 1988;32(3): 255–61.
82. Greer, S., et al. Psychological response to breast cancer and 15-year outcome. *Lancet* 1990;335:49–50 [letter].
83. Greer, S., et al. Adjuvant psychological therapy for patients with cancer: a prospective randomised trial. *BMJ* 1992;304: 675–80.
84. Grossarth-Maticek, R., and H. J. Eysenck. Length of survival and lymphocyte percentage in women with mammary cancer as a function of psychotherapy. *Psycholog Rep* 1989;65:315–21.

85. Fawzy, F. I., et al. A structured psychiatric intervention for cancer patients. II. Changes over time in immunological measures. *Arch Gen Psychiatr* 1990;47:729–35.

86. Derogatis, L. R., et al. Psychological coping mechanisms and survival time in metastatic breast cancer. *JAMA* 1979;242(14):1504–8.

87. Bridge, L. R., et al. Relaxation and imagery in the treatment of breast cancer. *BMJ* 1988;297:1169–71.

88. Simonton, O. C., et al. *Getting well again.* Bantam Books, New York, 1982.

89. Spiegel, D., et al. Effects of psychosocial treatment on survival of patients with metastatic breast cancer. *Lancet* 1989;ii:888–91.

90. Simonton, O. C., and S. Mathews-Simonton. Cancer and stress—counselling the cancer patient. *Med J Aust* 1981;1:679–83.

91. Siegel, B. *Love, medicine, and miracles.* Harper & Row, New York, 1986.

92. Spiegel, D., et al. Effects of psychosocial treatment on survival of patients with metastatic breast cancer. *Lancet* 1989;ii:888–91.

93. Simonton, O. C., and S. Mathews-Simonton. Cancer and stress — counselling the cancer patient. *Med J Aust* 1981;1:679–83.

94. Bridge, L. R., et al. Relaxation and imagery in the treatment of breast cancer. *BMJ* 1988;297:1169–71.

95. Greer, S., et al. Psychological response to breast cancer: effect on outcome. *Lancet* 1979;ii:785–7.

96. Pettingal, K. W., S. Greer, et al. Mental attitudes to cancer: an additional prognostic factor. *Lancet* 1985;i:750 [letter].

97. Greer, S., et al. Psychological response to breast cancer and 15-year outcome. *Lancet* 1990;335:49–50 [letter].

98. Grossarth-Maticek, R., and H. J. Eysenck. Length of survival and lymphocyte percentage in women with mammary cancer as a function of psychotherapy. *Psycholog Rep* 1989;65:315–21.

99. Mae, E. *How I conquered cancer naturally.* Production House, San Diego, 1975.

100. Cassileth, B. R., et al. Survival and quality of life among patients receiving unproven as compared with conventional cancer therapy. *N Engl J Med* 1991;324:1180–5.

101. Moss, R. W. *Cancer therapy: the independent consumer's guide to nontoxic treatment and prevention.* Equinox Press, New York, 1992.

102. Walters, R. *Options: the alternative cancer therapy book.* Avery Publishing, Garden City Park, NY, 1993.

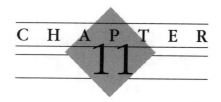

My Alternative Treatment Decisions

CATHY

Having opted for limited surgery and declined radiation and chemotherapy, my question was what to do next. Like many women with early-stage breast cancer, I hoped that the surgery was enough. But I couldn't know that. I turned to alternative medicine to explore other options.

Boosting immunity is the core of my alternative approach. The immune system requires strong natural killer cell activity to destroy cancer cells, and natural killer cell activity has been found to be an important predictor of cancer prognosis. Depression and inadequate social support reduce natural killer cell activity.[1]

After my diagnosis, despite strong support from friends and family, I was depressed, and it frightened me. I knew the depression might impair my immune system, which I couldn't afford — yet another depressing thought! But as Steve pointed out in the previous chapter, research has also shown that psychological intervention can help. Because psychological factors can affect natural killer cell activity,[2] I felt that dealing with my feelings through counseling might *boost* my immunity. And I was especially hopeful after learning that psychological intervention has doubled life expectancy with late-stage breast cancer patients,[3] as it has with other cancer patients.[4] Perhaps even more dramatic results might be possible for early-stage patients. So I dove into the deep end of the pool. Within a week of diagnosis I started individual counseling sessions (see Chapter 4). This support gave me the courage to explore other psychological options.

I met with a colleague and friend who had trained with the Simontons (see Chapter 10), and we talked about using imagery to fight the cancer. She suggested that I not get caught up in "doing it right." This turned out to be good advice, as I tend to obsess about the "right" way rather than finding what fits for me. Rather, she suggested, I should simply get the best therapist I could find (which I had already done). She recommended letting the imagery emerge naturally.

While I waited for that to happen, I also wanted to do more; the idea of joining a support group appealed to me. Most support groups in Portland at that time were in hospital settings, aimed largely at mastectomy patients (more options are now available). Nevertheless, one group captured my attention. It was an imaging group, and I attended it weekly until it ended nine months later.

The group provided an amazing experience. Every week the leader guided us on a journey into our imaginations. His imagery took us to the mountains or to the beach and used the healing power of the sun. It was generally a forty-five-minute "trip" that was deeply relaxing. He taped the sessions and encouraged us to borrow the tapes. When he suggested listening three times a day, I resisted — I felt I couldn't spare the time when I was already involved in other time-consuming treatments. However, I pushed myself to do it.

Within three days my body and spirit could feel the benefit through a release of physical tension. When I'm stressed or frightened, I tighten up, which affects my whole system, causing constipation, pulled muscles, etc. The stress wears on me and I get sluggish. By releasing the physical tension and the attendant side effects, I felt in charge of my body again. I could literally feel my powerlessness and depression transforming into hope and fighting spirit.

Subsequently, I read Steven Greer's research reporting that a patient's psychological response to breast cancer determined the outcome more than any other single factor (see Chapter 10). Patients with a "fighting spirit" had the best chance of survival.[5] Further research by this same group reported a patient's psychological response could be modified through counseling;[6] a "fighting spirit" could be nourished. I was beginning to discover this on my own through individual counseling and the imaging group. I knew something was changing; I could feel it in my body. And, as a typical American, I figured more might be better.

I found a professionally led support group (similar to Bernie Siegel's ECaP groups mentioned in Chapter 10), for people with chronic or life-threatening illnesses. I felt at home there because talking about alternative treatments was okay. When such talk had started in the imaging group at the hospital, a medical doctor had been brought in to quash it.

Because we were able to fully express ourselves in the new group, we quickly moved on to the real purpose of a support group — to explore our feelings about having cancer. I signed up for two ten-week series and would have done more had the group continued. Because I found meeting with other breast cancer survivors such a positive experience, I didn't stop there. Through Steve, I had met a psychologist who was also a breast cancer survivor, so I called her to ask if she might be interested in forming a mini-support group. We've been meeting monthly ever since and have become good friends. Sometimes we don't even mention cancer, but we both know it's always an option. We've shared doctor stories, cancer articles we've read, fears of a possible recurrence, and the thrill of celebrating yet another year of being healthy and living fully. My hope is that we'll still be getting together for lunch at 85; but, if either of us does have a recurrence, I know we'll be there for each other, and that knowledge is comforting.

From early on, I combined some of my psychological work with a naturopathic treatment called constitutional hydrotherapy.*

---

*Steve didn't talk about hydrotherapy in Chapter 10 because there's virtually no research linking it directly to the treatment of cancer. If you have a naturopathic doctor and you're interested in hydrotherapy, refer your doctor to the recent book on the subject: *Lectures in Naturopathic Hydrotherapy* by W. Boyle and A. Saine (Buckeye Naturopathic Press, East Palestine, Ohio, 1988). Do not do hydrotherapy without a doctor's guidance or use hot temperature over the affected breast.

It involves the use of hot and cold (water) packs to stimulate the immune system. Initially, it took an hour a day, four days a week for months. Steve administered the treatments. Even though it was time-consuming, I enjoyed this treatment.

By the time I started hydrotherapy, I had already started going to the imagery group, so I combined the two therapies. On the advice of my Simonton-trained friend, I'd altered the guided imagery to fit my own needs. For example, the group leader had advised us to do the guided imagery sitting up, but I found lying on the bed with my cat, Bessie, worked better for me. While listening to the guided imagery tapes, with Steve administering hydrotherapy with a loving touch, I would go into a deep relaxation and come out of it truly refreshed.

During one of the early hydrotherapy sessions, an image came to me for fighting the cancer. I've always been drawn to nature and to reverential Native American stories of animals as spirits. I was lying on white sheets with white towels for hydrotherapy, listening to one of my relaxation tapes and thinking about fighting the cancer, when suddenly a picture of a polar bear came to me.

At a "New Age" book store, I had bought guided imagery tapes for cancer patients (see Appendix B). With the help of these tapes, my first image developed into an army of tiny white polar bears entering my bloodstream and searching for cancer. When they found cancer cells, the bears would dislodge them from healthy tissue with their claws. My polar bears would then eat the cancer cells, leaving me disease-free. In an effort to enhance my imagery, I would visit the polar bear exhibit at the zoo to watch them eating and playing. I noticed how delicately they scooped up the herring, and I imagined my cancer cells as dead herring that could be deftly extricated from healthy tissue. This powerful image suited me well. I had two private sessions with the guided imagery group leader to create special tapes designed around my polar bears. I liked the timbre of his voice and associated it with the healing I felt in his group.

Much later, at a symposium on healing and the mind, I saw slides of natural killer cells. I was amazed. They looked like white puffs of fur — my miniature polar bears.

Because I had shared my polar bear imagery with those close to me, friends gave me beautiful polar bear figures which stand on my dresser and refrigerator to this day. Others sent polar bear greeting cards that are still taped to the inside of the cupboard holding my vitamins and herbs. The bears and cards are a steady reminder of the love that sent them to me. What could be more healing?

Taped beside the cards are fortune cookie maxims:

You will enjoy good health.

You will enjoy good health and be surrounded by luxury.

It is good to know things are improving.

Good health will be yours for a long time.

Long life is in store for you.

I got most of these fortunes (many of them repeatedly) during the first year after my diagnosis. They always made my day! I look at my polar bear pictures and glance at my fortunes every time I take herbs or vitamins.

And I take *lots* of vitamins: vitamin C, beta-carotene, selenium, vitamin E, and a multivitamin (see Chapter 13). I also take many herbs: an equivalent of the Hoxsey formula, taheebo (pau d'arco or lapacho), chaparral, goldenseal (*Hydrastis*), poke root (*Phytolacca*), and mistletoe (*Viscum album*). I also take a thymus extract to boost immune function.*

---

*Steve didn't discuss most of these treatments because they are fairly obscure compared with laetrile, shark cartilage, etc. In addition, he felt the level of scientific support is either insufficient or contradictory. For example, goldenseal, poke root, and thymus appear to boost immune function, and the scientific support for thymus extracts is both clear and consistent. Yet work with cancer patients is almost nonexistent for poke root and goldenseal, and cancer research is inconsistent and contradictory for thymus extracts. Moreover, the thymus research has been done with special products quite different from thymus pills found in the health food store. If you want to read more, see Ralph Moss's *Cancer Therapy* (Equinox Press, Garden City Park, NY, 1992). *Use these natural medicines and supplements only with the guidance of a doctor well-versed in their application, dosages, and potential toxicities.*

At the beginning, I took 50 pills a day. Now I'm down to a mere 35. Twelve are vitamin C. If you have trouble swallowing pills, vitamin C can easily be taken as a powder mixed with water. Normally, I don't have difficulty taking pills. Nevertheless, taking so many was an imposing task. My therapist suggested taking them meditatively in the spirit of healing. This helpful recommendation led me to develop a ritual around my pill swallowing rather than chug-a-lugging them to "get it over with."

My determination to heal body, mind, and spirit and prevent a recurrence didn't happen all at once; but it was a series of small steps. Initially, I was willing to do no more than read Bernie Siegel's book. The process evolved to include counseling, imagery, support groups, supplements, herbal medicine, hydrotherapy, diet and lifestyle changes. My biggest changes have been dietary. These modifications are directed at preventing a recurrence and are discussed in Chapter 15.

Remember, breast cancer is not melanoma. You have some time to make changes. You don't have to do everything all at once. Do whatever feels useful, possible, and reasonable to you. For instance, if you are a compulsive overeater, bulimic, or anorectic, trying to do dietary changes may be a setup for failure. Why not consider a change that feels possible? Then you can build on that victory. Any step toward healing and life is cause for celebration.

References

1. Levy, S., et al. Correlation of stress factors with sustained depression of natural killer cell activity and predicted prognosis in patients with breast cancer. *J Clin Oncol* 1987;5:348–53.

2. Levy, S., et al. Perceived social support and tumor estrogen/progesterone receptor status as predictors of natural killer cell activity in breast cancer patients. *Psychosomatic Med* 1990;52:73–85.

3. Spiegel, D., et al. Effect of psychosocial treatment on survival of patients with metastatic breast cancer. *Lancet* 1989;ii:888–91.

4. Simonton, O., and S. Matthews-Simonton. Cancer and stress — counselling the cancer patient. *Med J Aust* 1981;1:679–83.

5. Greer, S., et al. Psychological response to breast cancer and 15-year outcome. *Lancet* 1990;335:49–50.

6. Greer, S., et al. Adjuvant psychological therapy for patients with cancer: a prospective randomised trial. *BMJ* 1992;304:675–80.

PART 3

Preventing Breast Cancer

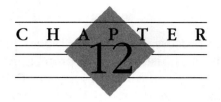

Diet and Prevention

STEVE

"Tell me what a culture eats and I'll tell you its breast cancer risk." This is what I say to my nutrition students. By the end of the course they can do the same thing, because the big picture is surprisingly simple. Traditional Oriental diets are associated with a very low breast cancer risk, traditional Mediterranean diets with an intermediate risk, and Western diets with a very high breast cancer risk.

But determining which overall diets cause or protect against breast cancer is not the top priority of scientists. Often, they seem to be looking for specific factors — magic bullets — rather than at the big picture.

Broccoli is a good example. Researchers are now trying to prove that broccoli protects against cancer because of its sulforaphane content. But others say it must be the beta-carotene. Some feel the high level of vitamin C in broccoli may be responsible. Glucaric acid in broccoli has its advocates too, as does indole-3-carbinol. Who knows? It could be the fiber. Researchers are keeping busy looking for the magic bullet when they already have a veritable assault rifle to use against cancer. Attempts to attribute its effects to any one ingredient miss the boat; such efforts don't necessarily even constitute good science. Perhaps it just doesn't sound intellectual enough to say "Eat broccoli — it's good for you," though that may well be what we need to hear.

Reviewing the research will require taking a long look at the reductionistic hunt for magic bullets. That's what's out there. But I hope that, in the process, you'll see a bigger picture emerging. Vegetables, fruit, and fish provide protection. Beans, whole grains, nonfat yogurt, and olive oil are fine. Other nonfat dairy products are okay in moderation. But most of the rest of the American diet is linked with trouble.

DIETARY FAT

For years researchers told us that a high-fat diet causes breast cancer. But in 1992, the large Nurses' Health Study group found no such link.[1] Published in the prestigious *Journal of the American Medical Association,* this report has received much attention.

Researchers have questioned the results,[2-5] but many reporters have accepted the report unconditionally. It's fun to believe ice cream doesn't hurt you. "Fat, the stuff that makes ice cream creamy and hamburgers juicy, now seems exonerated as a health risk for breast cancer."[6] "Recent studies have all but thrown out what had been the primary suspect: dietary fat."[7] Such positions distort the facts and are dangerous to the health of American women.

Correlation of Dietary Fat with Breast Cancer

Years ago, the fat intake of many countries was plotted on a graph against breast cancer rates.[8] A dramatic relationship emerged. With few exceptions, the more fat a society consumed per person, the higher the risk of breast cancer. Ten out of ten international studies looking at large differences in fat intake from one country to another found the relationship.[9] For travelers, this difference is obvious. In extremely low-risk countries like Thailand or South Korea, one sees slim women who eat remarkably little of the fat associated with breast cancer. In high-risk countries, like England and America, women eat diets high in animal fat and have higher body weight. Animal research supports this relationship; high-fat diets cause mammary cancer[10] — a fact known for more than half a century.[11]

How Does Dietary Fat Cause Breast Cancer?

The key to the relationship between fat and cancer is probably estrogen. Dietary fat increases body weight, increasing the size and, to some extent, the number of fat cells. Fat cells make estrogen, which promotes breast cancer. Therefore, more weight indirectly means more estrogen. There's little question that being overweight boosts the risk of postmenopausal breast cancer — the breast cancer we see so much of in societies where women consume high-fat diets.*

Excess weight from a high-fat diet also leads to an early first menstrual cycle in adolescent girls.[12] Each added menstrual cycle exposes the breast to high levels of estrogen.

Women who consume high levels of fat have, on average, higher levels of active estrogen.[13] Putting women on a low-fat diet reduces their estrogen levels.[14,15] All these pieces fit together.

But even before the Nurses' Health Study, the clear relationship between dietary fat and breast cancer began to fall apart with the publication of within-population studies.

When Is a "Low-Fat" Diet Not Low-Fat?

A within-population study looks at women from the same country or culture — that is, women from within a given population. Many within-population studies have looked for a link between fat intake and breast cancer risk. Some find it, but more don't.[16]

This is not surprising. Within a population, people eat basically the same diet. Nobody in Tibet has a BLT for lunch, and everyone in Newark knows what blue cheese dressing is. People who eat the same way don't exhibit much variation in fat intake. At the top end of the typical American range, we eat over 40 percent of our calories from fat. But the bottom end of our range, well over 30 percent calories from fat, is still considered a high-fat

---

*Premenopausal breast cancer rates vary relatively little between high- and low-fat societies. We don't know why. Details about estrogen, body weight, and breast cancer risk are covered in Chapter 14.

diet. Finding variations in breast cancer risk between high-fat and even higher fat diets is difficult. Real differences might exist, but they may be obscured by other issues.

The statistics on high-fat versus higher-fat studies can be compared to automobile accident survival rates. Your chance of surviving a collision is tied less to whether you go 80 mph versus 85 mph than to whether your seat belt is on. In the same way a car wreck is affected by factors other than speed, breast cancer is affected by factors other than fat. Some breast cancer risk factors are totally independent of diet — for example, remaining childless or carrying a predisposing gene. Just as differences in auto accident survival rates due to speed variations are insignificant compared to differences in survival rates determined by seat belt use, a combination of factors independent of fat can obscure variations in breast cancer risk that result from small differences between different high-fat diets. Driving 80 miles per hour isn't necessarily safe. Eating 35 percent of your calories from fat isn't safe either. Virtually all Americans eat too much fat, and a little more or less barely makes a difference.

When Is a Low-Fat Diet Really Low-Fat?

People in countries with extremely low breast cancer rates always get less than 25 percent of their calories from fat. And countries with breast cancer rates even higher than ours always get more than 35 percent — often more than 40 percent. Whenever scientists look at levels of fat intake that vary significantly from one country to the next, they see differences in postmenopausal breast cancer risk.

Many researchers believe that cutting fat intake will not help substantially until levels get down to 20 percent. Americans would have to cut their fat intake in half to go that low. Maureen Henderson of the Fred Hutchinson Cancer Research Center in Seattle has estimated that such a reduction would lower breast cancer rates for women between 55 and 69 years of age by 61 percent.[17] Then we'd be talking low-fat.

A Needle in a Haystack

Other factors also interfere with attempts to link fat and breast cancer within a population. Most studies depend on memories. People who really cut fat intake are not necessarily the same as those who write down that they cut fat intake. The women in these studies are not carefully monitored; no one is looking over their shoulders at the dinner table. We must rely on what they think they eat. Even conscientious participants may seriously underestimate their fat intake. So it's difficult to prove dietary fat causes breast cancer by studying a group of American women all eating a similar high-fat diet and all trying to remember just what it was they ate.

Maybe a Low-Fat Diet Just Protects Kids

If dietary fat influences the age of menarche (first menstrual cycle), maybe the only people who can lower their risk by cutting fat intake are preadolescents. Through diet, they can still postpone their first menstrual cycle and, therefore, delay their exposure to estrogen. If a low-fat diet is advantageous only to girls, it may be pointless to study fat intakes in adult women. Researchers have yet to sort this out.

But you are no longer preadolescent. Why should you switch to a low-fat diet if you're too old to be helped by it?

Some evidence suggests the situation is not that discouraging or that simple. Women in Japan who get breast cancer have better survival rates than do their American counterparts,[18] particularly with postmenopausal breast cancer[19] — the breast cancer associated with high-fat diets. The difference between Japanese and American risks has nothing to do with genes. Japanese American women eating an American diet have a much higher risk than do women in Japan.[20] The only relevant thing Japanese women do differently than Americans as adults, as far as researchers can tell, is maintain their low-fat diet. Japanese adult women who have recently migrated from Japan have an increased risk of breast cancer.[21] This finding is supported by another report showing that Asian women (including Japanese) who migrate to America in their early thirties have the same risk as those who migrate before their first menstrual cycle. The authors say "there was no direct evidence of an especially susceptible period, during either menarche or early reproductive life."[22] If switching away from a very low-fat diet as an adult can increase risk, it seems plausible that switching to a very low-fat diet as an adult should reduce risk. So perhaps changing dietary fat as an adult is important. "Perhaps not," some medical doctors might say. And they're right — we're not sure. But what's the worst that can happen if you decide to eat like people who rarely get breast cancer? It won't be the end of the world — you'll have to learn new eating habits and perhaps spend a little extra money for more exotic food. But what if such a change saves your life? Until more is known, I believe it makes perfect sense to emulate the lifestyle of countries where women rarely get breast cancer. Highly respected researchers from the American Health Foundation agree with this premise.[23]

Reducing fat may be helpful in preventing breast cancer to begin with (primary prevention) or in preventing a recurrence (secondary prevention). (See Chapter 13 for more information about primary versus secondary prevention.) Swedish researchers have recently discovered that a low-fat diet translates into lower risk of a recurrence for women who are estrogen receptor positive (see Chapter 9).[24] Researchers from the University of Hawaii have found that high-fat diets in breast cancer patients increase the risk of death.[25]

Effect of the Nurses' Health Study

Recall that the Nurses' Health Study found no link between fat intake and breast cancer. As we see in Chapters 13 and 14, the study was also unable to verify most of the other dietary and lifestyle risk factors that have been identified by many researchers. Why?

To their credit, the Nurses' Health Study staff realized they needed to find women whose fat intake was below the average range. Initially these researchers divided their subjects into five groups on the basis of fat intake; but even the group with the lowest fat intake ate a high-fat diet. So they cut the subjects into ten groups of equal size on the basis of fat intake. The 10 percent eating the lowest level of fat claimed to eat a diet analyzed to be "less than 29 percent" of calories from fat — significantly higher than the 20 percent many researchers believe to be the beginning of protection. When the group eating less than 29 percent fat was compared with those eating higher levels of fat, no hint of a relationship to breast cancer risk was found. Because the Nurses' Health Study asked women about their diets before they were diagnosed (a "prospective" study), most problems associated with memory were eliminated. But the researchers failed to consider fat intake during childhood and, more significantly, they failed to look at women with a fat intake averaging less than 20 percent.

The Nurses' Health Study report was big and expensive. The principal researchers came from Harvard. It was published in the *Journal of the American Medical Association*. And it came up completely empty-handed. For these reasons, the results were given enormous weight in the research community and elsewhere. But another factor played a critical role in acceptance of the results of this study: Many medical doctors assume that if less than 29 percent fat doesn't work, there's no point in looking further. They don't believe you will be willing to eat less than 29 percent of your calories from fat. They are wrong.

John McDougall, who developed the low-fat vegetarian McDougall Diet, reported an attempt to dramatically reduce dietary fat in five postmenopausal women with a history of breast cancer.[26] All five stayed on the diet, eating only 8 percent calories from fat during a three-month experiment. Both estrogen and prolactin (another hormone associated with breast cancer promotion) dropped more than 36 percent.

Researchers from the Ontario Cancer Institute in Toronto have attempted to encourage women to dramatically reduce dietary fat. At four months, women who were randomly assigned to the low-fat group were eating an average of 22 percent fat. When they were followed for two years, 60 percent of the women in the low-fat group were eating 20 percent calories from fat or less and 80 percent were eating 25 percent fat or less.[27] Other studies have also proven that dramatic drops in dietary fat are possible and are accompanied by decreased estrogen levels.[28,29]

Rather than stimulating lively debate, the Nurses' Health Study has put the lid on it. To make matters worse, the researchers have overstated their case. They say, for example, "Little or no association between fat intake and breast cancer has been seen in most epidemiologic studies." To support this faulty claim they cite a review article by Goodwin and Boyd. But Goodwin and Boyd say, "The majority of the epidemiologic evidence is consistent with a causal association between dietary fat and breast cancer risk."[30]

Most of the research does find a correlation between fat and breast cancer — including a handful of within-population studies. It just hasn't received as much press as the Nurses' Health Study. For example, the data from twelve different within-population trials were pooled by Geoffrey Howe from the University of Toronto and a group of international researchers. Of the individual trials in this study, some found that fat was associated very clearly with increased risk[31] while others reported fat made no difference.[32] But when all the numbers were put together, providing a better look at the true relationship between fat and breast cancer, the analysis showed "a consistent, statistically significant, positive association between breast cancer risk and saturated fat intake in postmenopausal women."[33] The 20 percent who ate the most fat had almost a 46 percent increased breast cancer risk compared with those eating the least fat. This relationship was found even though at least one of the twelve studies probably *could not* have shown a correlation: A Greek study reported "no association" with total fat;[34] but Greek women consume much of their fat from olive oil. As we see later in this chapter, olive oil does not cause breast cancer.

Howe published a review showing that three of four other studies using the same research design as the Nurses' Health Study did find that a high-fat diet caused breast cancer,[35] including Howe's own work.[36] Subsequently, two out of three additional studies using the same design have also succeeded in finding a relation between fat and breast cancer.[37,38,39] And even the authors of the Nurses' Study tell people to eat a low-fat diet to reduce their risk of colon cancer.

But, ignoring the results of the Nurses' Health Study would be as unfair as is the current trend toward discounting most of the other research. The Nurses' Health Study has proven something: It's useless for adult women to moderately cut back their dietary fat. This is not to say that moderate changes in your preadolescent daughter or granddaughter's diet would necessarily be a waste of time. But if you make moderate changes to your diet, you will not reduce your risk. This bad news — and there's no other way to describe it — must be viewed in perspective.

If we focus on your dietary fat, two possibilities exist: Either it's too late (as an adult) to have a low-fat diet reduce your risk, or you need to dramatically decrease dietary fat before your risk will decline. We don't know which of these two hypotheses is true, though I believe the Japanese research mentioned earlier favors the second hypothesis. Cathy's trial with a radical reduction in fat remains an experiment — but one that offers considerable hope.

Is It Fat, or Is It Just Calories?

A recent California trial followed 590 women for fifteen years until fifteen cases of breast cancer developed. These fifteen women ate more of every possible type of fat than did the women who remained cancer-free, but an even stronger correlation was found between *high calories* and high breast cancer risk.[40] Animal research has clearly shown that a high-calorie diet increases mammary cancer risk even when the amount of dietary fat stays the same.[41] As a result, some researchers have suggested that fat isn't the problem — it's the calories.[42]

This argument is shortsighted and not supported by the data. One review of the literature shows that the correlation between dietary fat and breast cancer is considerably stronger than the association between calories and breast cancer.[43] Of course, fat is loaded with calories — ounce for ounce it has far more calories than anything else. In rats, special diets can be created with few calories on the one hand, but a high percentage of calories coming from fat on the other. In real life, however, making a distinction between fat and calories has no meaning. All low-fat diets are low in calories. All high-calorie diets are loaded with fat.

If it were true that calories, rather than fats, were related to breast cancer, then all types of fats would be associated with an equal breast cancer risk because they all have the same number of calories. But as we shall see later in this chapter, certain types of fats do not cause breast cancer and might even reduce the risk. As far back as 1945 some cancer researchers knew that fat was not merely a synonym for calories.[44]

I'm not saying that women eating more calories don't have a higher risk of cancer. They do. But for practical purposes, if you cut out most of your dietary fat, the calories come way down. It can't go any other way. However, even independent of its high caloric content, certain fats are linked with cancer.

Is It Fat, or Is It More Complicated?

By focusing on a magic bullet — fat — we have ignored the big picture. The key is not just the potential magic bullet called fat. But it is clearly related to diet. Virtually all researchers acknowledge that. Wherever people eat junk food, cookies, candy, red meat, fried food, processed food, etc., breast cancer rates are high. Wherever people eat mostly grains and vegetables plus fruit and fish, the risk is low. Our breast cancer rate is more than eight times as high as the rate in Korea and twenty-two times that of Thailand.[45] If we know what kind of diet is associated with protection and what kind of diet causes trouble, why not switch rather than fight?

I'm less concerned with why oriental diets lead to less breast cancer than I am with the undeniable fact that they do. For Cathy and me, sashimi tastes better than fish and chips, Thai curried vegetables beat macaroni and cheese, and Vietnamese salad rolls are more exotic than sausage. We're not suffering with these changes — we're only paying more. But think what it costs to treat a breast cancer recurrence.

At one point, Cathy and I were in the office of a surgeon who was shocked to discover Cathy had had only some of the treatments suggested by conventional medicine. "Just what are you doing?" she asked Cathy. "Since the surgery I've been living like women do who don't get breast cancer," Cathy replied. "We don't believe in that," the surgeon said. I laughed at her honesty.

What she meant was that once the usual therapies are given, conventional medicine "believes" in waiting . . . for the breast cancer to return, saying dietary changes haven't yet been totally *proven* to reduce risk. Although it's true that we're not sure exactly which dietary factors are most important — fat levels, fiber, antioxidants, or other factors yet to be discovered — we do know that oriental diets lead to a much lower risk.

Don't lose sight of the basics. All countries consuming lots of meat, dairy, and processed fatty foods have a high risk. All who eat primarily vegetables, grains, and fish have a low risk. Remembering this simple distinction will keep us clear of the mental baggage acquired by so many research groups all hunting for the magic bullet that determines risk.

If you are agonizing about whether to cut your dietary fat, here's one piece of good news. Certain types of fat need not be excluded. This makes the dietary changes much easier. It also means you don't really need to cut your dietary fat to less than 20 percent of calories — you just need to stop eating certain fats.

Safe Fat

Fat tastes good. That's why we eat so much of it.

Fortunately, two sources of fat don't cause breast cancer, and at least one of them may well reduce your risk. Fish-eating countries have lower breast cancer rates.[46] Feeding fish oil to animals reduces mammary cancer.[47,48] And women who eat fish have a lower risk than women who don't.[49] There's no need to restrict fish, including fatty fish, unless you need to lose weight. High-fat fish include mackerel, salmon, herring, black cod (sable fish), sardines, and anchovies. If you like sardines, look for those packed in mustard, tomato sauce, sild sardine oil, water, or olive oil.

If you are not overweight, eat fish as frequently as you like. The type of oil in fish is distinctly different from that in bacon, steak, fried chicken, or cheese fat. Fish oil interferes with the production of a hormonelike substance called prostaglandin E₂, or PGE₂ for short. Breast cancer patients make too much PGE₂, which is an immune system culprit, responsible for the inability of breast cancer patients to kill their cancer cells.[50]

Some vegetarians avoid fish for ethical reasons. Of course, this is an individual choice. But it's important to separate ethical concerns from health issues. There is no scientific support for the idea that breast cancer patients should avoid fish and every reason to believe they should be encouraged to eat it.

The other safe fat is olive oil. Olive oil and its major component, oleic acid, do not have the same cancer-promoting effects that other common vegetable oils show in animal studies,[51,52,53] nor do they interfere with immune function as other fats do.[54] Populations consuming high levels of olive oil have relatively low breast cancer risks.[55] Olive oil intake is associated with decreases in overall death rates.[56] Unless you need to lose weight, olive oil is good for you.

Oleic acid, on the other hand, has sometimes correlated with a higher risk of breast cancer.[57] But when that occurs, the source of oleic acid is inevitably not olive oil. Meat and other foods linked to cancer contain some oleic acid. Links between non-olive-oil sources of oleic acid and cancer therefore reflect dietary problems unrelated to olive oil.

It is not clear that olive oil actually reduces cancer risks the way fish oil does. Nonetheless, there is little reason to restrict its use unless you're watching calories.

Knowing Your Olive Oil

Olive oil comes in three forms. Some olive oil is labeled "pure." Surprisingly, this means the oil has been extracted with chemicals. For the purist, therefore, "pure" is impure.

The second grade of olive oil is labeled "virgin." Unlike "pure" olive oil, virgin olive oil has only been pressed.

The top of the line is called "extra virgin." One of my students asked if this means no one even pressed the olives. The true definition of "extra virgin" is technical. Like virgin olive oil, extra virgin results from pressing olives. After the oil has been extracted, measurements are made to see if the small chains of fat (primarily oleic acid) are tied up in little packages of three. If virtually all the oleic acid is in these small bundles, the manufacturer can label the oil "extra virgin." But if a sizable amount of the oleic acid is free, the word "extra" cannot be used.

A higher content of free oleic acid impairs the flavor of the oil. More importantly, there appears to be some increase in cancer risk associated with free oleic acid in some animal studies. Why this occurs is unclear, but free oleic acid can be avoided simply by using extra virgin olive oil.

How About Canola Oil — The Poor Woman's Olive Oil?

Canola oil is considered an olive oil substitute because, next to olive oil, canola has the highest level of oleic acid, but the two oils are not the same. We know almost nothing about canola oil and cancer risk. Therefore, until more research has been done, I suggest sticking with olive oil.

Cooking with Olive Oil

Because olive oil smokes at fairly low heating temperatures, it doesn't work well for wok (or any high-temperature) cooking. Olive oil works fine for sautéing as long as you keep the temperature down.

Unlike most refined vegetable oils, olive oil imparts its characteristic flavor and odor to food. People in the Middle East or southern Europe find the flavor and aroma to be big pluses. For some Americans, however, olive oil initially seems odd. Stick with it. After a while you may come to enjoy the taste as much as the Greeks and Lebanese do. Initially, I had difficulty with olive-oil-cooked oriental dishes. With homemade Chinese or Thai food, I now add a few drops of oriental sesame oil to the pan along with olive oil. Oriental sesame oil is not the same as standard sesame oil. It's darker in color, costs more, is found in the oriental section of the supermarket, and smells like toasted sesame seeds. Just a few drops will overpower the flavor of olive oil, giving a dish an oriental flavor.

What If You Need to Count Calories?

For sautéing, you can use either Teflon with no oil or spray a fine mist of olive oil on the pan. (Several companies now sell olive oil in spray cans; it's usually not extra virgin, but the amount used can be so small that it's hardly worth worrying about.) Calories can be dramatically reduced by using the spray instead of spoonfuls of oil. Spraying air-dried popcorn with just a bit of olive oil augments the otherwise bone-dry taste without the calories and saturated fat of butter.

Changing the Type of Fat in Your Diet

Animal fat from sources other than fish correlates more closely with breast cancer risk in humans than do any of the other fats.[58] Saturated fat, found primarily in dairy, beef, pork, eggs, and poultry, has been linked to an increased risk that breast cancer will spread to lymph nodes.[59] Saturated fat also correlates with elevated levels of prolactin, a breast-cancer-promoting hormone.[60] Some researchers find that meat correlates most directly with breast cancer risk.[61] Others find strong links with dairy fat[62] or eggs.[63] Some studies uncover multiple associations — with meat, cheese, and total saturated fat.[64]

Reducing animal fats by switching to leaner cuts, trimming visible fat, or substituting chicken, will still leave you with high-fat foods, albeit not quite as high. The question, then, is how can you completely avoid these foods?

Getting Rid of Dairy Fat

For many people, dairy fat is easy to eliminate. Whole milk can be replaced with nonfat milk. Nonfat yogurt can replace regular yogurt, and nonfat frozen yogurt can substitute for ice cream.

Why not just use 2 percent milk — isn't that lower than the 20 percent we've been talking about? NO — not close! So-called 2 percent milk gets more than a quarter of its calories from fat. So why is it called 2 percent? Milk is mostly water. If we take dried milk solids containing more than 25 percent calories from fat and add water, there's a point where the container will include only 2 percent fat by weight. But water has no calories, so its addition doesn't affect the proportion of calories coming from fat. More than 25 percent of the calories still comes from fat. But when we include the water, only 2 percent of the weight is fat. Just as pure olive oil is not pure, low-fat milk is not low-fat.

As you can now calculate, whole (3.5 to 4 percent) milk derives about half of its calories from fat. Why is it legal to call it 4 percent? For the same reason it's legal to call white bread "enriched." The dairy industry and large bakeries have clout in Washington. Both 4 percent milk and enriched white bread are distortions created to mislead the consumer into thinking such choices are healthful.

The Ins and Outs of Dairy Replacement

Replacing ice cream with nonfat frozen yogurt is simple. But when you add most of the available toppings, you're adding fat. And when you buy quarts of nonfat frozen yogurt in the health food store, read the label carefully. Often the yogurt is nonfat, but the added chocolate or nuts are anything but. Check the fruit flavors and try adding your own fresh fruit to supply flavor without additional fat.

Nonfat frozen yogurt cannot yet match ice cream in what food processors call "mouth feel," but it's getting closer. When you bite into high-fat ice cream, it almost bites you back. If you've encountered only the kind of frozen yogurt that tastes like plastic, keep trying. I recently sampled some by Alta Dena that tasted so much like ice cream I'm still not sure I didn't get ice cream by mistake. But it's best to save nonfat frozen yogurt as an occasional treat. Sugar levels of frozen yogurt are usually sky high. As noted earlier, calories correlate with breast cancer and, as we'll see, so apparently does sugar.*

Butter should not be replaced with margarine because, like butter, margarine is almost solid fat. As naturopathic doctors had long suspected, margarine was recently implicated in causing heart disease (a finding shared even by the Nurses' Health Study group),[65] and fats from margarine have reduced cancer survival time in animals.[66]

The key to eliminating butter is not a butter substitute, but a change in the foods that go with butter. Cathy discusses her solutions in Chapter 15. You might consider switching away from eating so much bread if you're used to buttering it. For example, rice tastes fine without butter. If you need butter on white potatoes, switch to sweet potatoes or yams, or try using nonfat yogurt or olive oil. Really fresh corn doesn't demand butter. When regular corn isn't fresh, hunt for white corn — it's often sweeter.

Nonfat cheese is becoming available in health food stores and supermarkets and, although it doesn't yet taste like the real thing, some brands are getting close. Don't overdo the nonfat cheese or milk, though. Some researchers are concerned that dairy links to cancer are not due to fat alone. Correlations between animal *protein* and breast cancer risks have been reported.[67,68,69] The animal protein and cancer association has not been intensively investigated. But if it holds up, even nonfat milk and cheese should be restricted. The question is, How?

Milk is hardest to avoid at breakfast. Try oatmeal without milk, or try oat bran with fruit or even fruit and nonfat yogurt. Nonfat yogurt has animal protein; but for reasons we don't under-

---

*Ounce for ounce, sugar has many fewer calories than fat. Nonetheless, because sugar does not have the fiber and noncaloric fillers that whole foods have, it is still quite high in calories.

stand, cultured dairy products (yogurt in particular) are not linked with cancer. In fact, yogurt is associated with protection.[70,71]

Fish can replace cheese as a protein source, although it may not work with fondue. Be creative. See Cathy's pizza recipe in Chapter 15.

How about calcium — won't restricting dairy products cause a problem? Nonfat yogurt has even more calcium than regular yogurt. (The lack of fat leaves room in the yogurt container for more of all the contents of yogurt *except* fat — including calcium.) Sardines are high in calcium as long as you eat the bones. Although many medical doctors suggest avoiding calcium pills, there's no reason to do so. It won't hurt to add 500 milligrams of calcium by pill. The only side effect is theoretical: Although the risk of kidney stones actually goes down for most people when they supplement their diet with calcium,[72] in theory a few patients with a tendency to form kidney stones might still be better off without calcium supplements. If you have a history of kidney stones, ask your nutrition-oriented doctor about the advisability of calcium supplements.

Saying Good-bye to Eggs

Whenever a recipe calls for an egg, use egg whites instead. The white of the egg is almost fat-free. For pancakes, Arrowhead Mills has a multigrain mix that tastes great without adding eggs or oil. Just spray the pan with a tiny bit of olive oil to keep the pancakes from sticking. Most bread and some pasta are egg-free. Read the labels. For breakfast, see the suggestions in the dairy discussion.

Eliminating Red Meat and Poultry

Changing your diet so that you eat vegetarian and fish foods only is much easier than giving up cigarettes. You can do it. Here are some tips.

Meat can be replaced with fish. Most meat-free recipes in Thai and Japanese cookbooks are fine. Vegetarian cookbooks are often helpful, but watch out for the cheese. Books on achieving a low-fat diet, such as those by Dean Ornish, John McDougall, and others, are now readily available and include recipes (see Appendix A). Most of these authors have a fetish about eliminating fat — even fat not associated with health problems. Remember, when it comes to breast cancer, you needn't be quite so restrictive. Add fish and olive oil as you like. Don't be put off; books advocating a nearly fat-free diet are geared to reducing heart attacks and not cancer. The same diet works for both. Societies with low rates of breast cancer have low rates of heart disease. Countries with high rates of heart disease have high breast cancer rates as well.[73]

Processed Food and Low-Fat Diets

Processed food used to be entirely off-limits on a low-fat diet, but not anymore. Several companies now sell baked (not fried) corn chips that are great with salsa. Although they are high in sugar, fat-free mayonnaise and salad dressing are now available. (Watch out for the words *light* or *lite* — they often signify reduced fat, not no fat.) Supermarkets carry old-fashioned rye crackers, and fat-free crackers are available in health food stores. Fat-free cookies are fine on occasion; but, as with frozen yogurt, don't make them a regular habit. They're loaded with sugar, which is associated with breast cancer risk in several studies.[74] "No sugar — fruit juice sweetened" on the label doesn't mean a product is any healthier than if the sugar were extracted from cane or sugar beets. Even my nutrition students sometimes act as if white sugar were made in poison gas factories and "fruit juice sweetened" were the same as picking fresh apples off a tree. Basically, sugar is sugar. The fiber is eliminated when white sugar or fruit juice concentrate is made. Fiber-depleted foods lose most of their value and all of their ability to protect us from the harmful effects of the sugar they often contain.

If you're not sure about a processed food, read the label, looking for fat. New fat-free foods are generally labeled as such in bold letters. Remember, the label "low-fat" does not usually signify no fat. It must say "fat-free." If a processed food has zero grams of fat per portion but "mono- and diglycerides" (fats) are on the label, it means that the amount of fat added is truly negligible.

Restaurants

Standard American restaurant fare presents a challenge. After all, it represents the same Western diet that got us into this mess in the first place. Baked or poached fish are sometimes available. Baked potatoes can also be ordered without butter or sour cream. Try adding olive oil. On request, vegetables can usually be cooked without butter.

Salad bars can be surprisingly difficult. Most dressings are high in fat. Olive oil and vinegar are often available, or you can bring a small container of fat-free dressing in your purse. Avoid the croutons, potato salad, coleslaw, imitation bacon, and other prepared foods that look or taste fatty — they usually are. Mayonnaise at a salad bar is rarely fat-free.

Cheap fish joints won't work. When fish is of poor quality, it has to be deep-fat-fried to disguise the taste. But many seafood restaurants do fit easily into a low-fat diet. Don't be concerned about fatty fish unless you need to count calories. Say "no butter, please." Have the fish baked, boiled, broiled, or poached.

In oriental restaurants, eat the vegetable and fish dishes. Forget the luncheon specials, which almost invariably contain some meat. Stay away from fried food; obviously, it's high in fat.

In Japanese restaurants, avoid sukiyaki (which contains beef) and tempura (which is deep-fat-fried). Virtually all other dishes on the menu are either very low in fat or contain only fatty fish. Don't feel guilty about splurging at the sushi bar. Tell yourself it's for medicinal purposes.

Most Italian restaurants offer pasta dishes with a meatless tomato-based sauce. Pesto sauce is okay if cheese has not been added to the mix. Ask. (Cathy has started growing her own basil so we can have homemade, inexpensive, cheese-free pesto.)

Middle Eastern food usually fits with the diet, because most of the fat comes from olive oil. But avoid lamb dishes, and see if the restaurant will bake the falafel rather than fry it. Tabouli, hummus, baba ghanoush, and pita bread are all fine.

Even though much of it is vegetarian, Indian food is difficult on the low-fat diet because it contains oil or ghee (clarified butter). Call ahead. Some Indian restaurants can substitute olive oil, but many won't.

Mexican restaurants are a challenge because the food is usually cooked in lard, and almost all meatless dishes have cheese. In the Northwest, we have Macheesmo Mouse — a chain of health-food Mexican restaurants that avoids lard. Whole wheat tortillas are available, and they'll leave off the cheese when asked. If you aren't lucky enough to find such an alternative, you may be able to put together your own soft tacos with plain tortillas, salad, salsa, and shrimp.

Traditional French food is high in fat, but some nouvelle cuisine dishes are catered to low-fat diets — ask. The easiest way to convey what you need is to say you're vegetarian, you don't eat eggs or dairy products (including butter), but you do eat fish.

How About Other Types of Fat?

If olive oil and fish are okay, and dairy, poultry, and red meat are not, what about vegetable oil, nuts, avocados, seeds, etc.? I was hoping you wouldn't ask.

These "polyunsaturated" fats cause mammary cancer in animals.[75] There is much less information about polyunsaturates and human cancer. In people, therefore, we're not so sure. Some researchers find a link.[76,77] Others don't.[78,79] Because these fats are carcinogenic in animals, Cathy generally avoids them. Small amounts of vegetable oils are used in most oriental dishes except in Japanese food. Several of these oriental countries have even lower breast cancer rates than Japan's. Cathy has chosen not to totally exclude oriental food sautéed in non-olive-based vegetable oil, though she avoids oriental vegetables that tend to soak up the oil (like eggplant dishes). At home, we stick with olive oil.

Nuts, seeds, and avocados also contain high amounts of polyunsaturates. Because of the animal studies and because of our ignorance regarding human cancer and these oils, Cathy severely restricts these foods. Three cashews on top of a low-fat oriental vegetarian dish, however, will not lead to disease. Each person needs to draw her own line.

Protecting Your Children and Grandchildren

If mice are placed on a high-fat diet while they are pregnant, the offspring will have more mammary cancer even if they are never fed a high-fat diet.[80] We're not sure why this happens. Nonetheless, if a woman is in her childbearing years, a low-fat diet might well protect her children. "There is no justification for high-fat diets during pregnancy," the principal investigator of the mouse study has said.[81]

Who Is Helped by the Low-Fat Diet?

If your preadolescent female family member severely restricts nonfish animal fat, her postmenopausal breast cancer risk will probably be reduced. At least in part this benefit is a result of postponing exposure to estrogen by delaying the menstrual cycle. If you are postmenopausal and you make the dietary switch, you may be buying some primary or secondary prevention as well. Recall that it's postmenopausal breast cancer that is tied to dietary fat. If you are premenopausal and have been diagnosed with breast cancer, it's unlikely that a high-fat diet caused your cancer. Cathy is still premenopausal. She eats the low-fat diet because she hopes to live long enough to become postmenopausal. When she does reach menopause, her risk of recurrence may be reduced as a result of cutting fat. Until then, it is not at all clear that her chances of a recurrence are affected by her low-fat diet. Menopause seemed a long way off when Cathy was diagnosed at age 43. But now that she's beyond five years of disease-free survival, the thought that her dietary diligence may be buying insurance for the very near future is comforting to both of us. I believe it makes sense for all women with breast cancer to think seriously about a low-fat diet.

Why Can't Tax Dollars Help Solve the Remaining Riddles?

The only way to prove that fat lowers human breast cancer is to do what is called an intervention trial. This means putting many women on a diet very low in fat and following the outcome for years.

In the early 1980s, the government-funded National Cancer Institute was about to sponsor the Women's Health Trial — an intervention trial using a diet with 20 percent of calories from fat. Skeptics felt women would not restrict themselves that much. But a feasibility study showed that the skeptics were wrong, as have successful attempts to get women on long-term very low-fat diets mentioned earlier in this chapter. Despite the success of the feasibility study, in 1988 the Women's Health Trial was derailed, officially because of finances, but potentially for reasons of medical politics, according to *Ms.* magazine.[82] Leading researchers have been asking for an intervention trial.[83,84,85] Recently, the National Institutes of Health launched the Women's Health Initiative, which will finally look at the effects of a long-term, low-fat diet on breast cancer risk. Nonetheless, the main thrust of federally funded breast cancer prevention research has shifted to tamoxifen in an attempt to reduce cancer incidence without violating conventional medicine's philosophical commitment to drugs, surgery and radiation. (In Chapter 9 the ongoing tamoxifen drug trial for breast cancer prevention is discussed in detail.)

Just Do It

It hasn't been proven that a thief will try to get into your house, but does that mean you shouldn't lock your door? Until we better understand how breast cancer works, a dramatic reduction in nonfish animal fat is as potentially important as is any other preventive tool now on the horizon.

Cathy has survived the diet. She even enjoys it. With rare exceptions,* I eat this way too, and I don't even have a life-threaten-

---

*I used to have occasional rich desserts in restaurants, but every time I did, one of my nutrition students miraculously appeared at the next table. Shame has eliminated my former indiscretions.

ing diagnosis hanging over my head. Yet. As I mentioned earlier, the low-fat diet protects against many diseases besides breast cancer. If you decide to dramatically reduce dietary fat, remember the lesson of the Nurses' Health Study — halfway measures will be to no avail. Just do it.

FIBER

Fiber comes from whole grains, fruits, vegetables, and beans. Most of it consists of sugar molecules linked together in a way that interferes with absorption of the sugar. But one type of fiber, lignan, looks and acts differently from all the others. Lignans resemble estrogen.

Lignan — Protective Fibers

Lignans are in seeds and whole grains. In the gut, bacteria transform these plant lignans into another form — sometimes confusingly called animal lignans — that can then be absorbed. Once absorbed, lignans interfere with estrogenic activity, acting somewhat like nature's tamoxifen but without the risks.[86]

Breast cancer patients excrete lower levels of urinary lignans than healthy women do.[87] The lack of sufficient lignan in the urine of breast cancer patients is due in part to a low-fiber diet. If you eat less plant lignan, you'll have less animal lignan to excrete in urine (and less circulating in your body to protect you against breast cancer).

Vegetarians eat more fiber (including lignan) than do non-vegetarians. Therefore, vegetarians excrete a high level of lignan. Vegetarian women who eat no dairy fat or eggs excrete far more lignan than do other vegetarians.[88]

Eating more cereals, whole grains, and seeds will increase your lignan intake somewhat. But by far the best source of lignan is flaxseed, which is sold in health food stores. Flaxseeds should be ground to make the lignan more absorbable. This should be done just before eating them to avoid rancidity. Flaxseeds are crunchy and have a mild flavor. A salad or sautéed vegetables won't suffer from their inclusion. Two teaspoons of ground flaxseeds can also be added to oatmeal or other cereals. (Avoid higher amounts, which can interfere with the body's ability to use vitamin B6.)

Animal and human studies support the protective effect of fiber. Rats put on a high-fiber diet develop fewer mammary tumors.[89] Cereal (grain) products have been linked with breast cancer protection. A Dutch study divided women into four equal groups (quartiles) on the basis of grain intake. The quartile eating the most grains had less than half the breast cancer risk of those eating the least.[90]

Earlier in this chapter, I mentioned the work of Geoffrey Howe, a researcher who, with others, combined the results of twelve studies and found a link between fat and breast cancer. The Howe report also looked at dietary fiber.[91] Women were divided into five equal groups (quintiles) on the basis of fiber intake. The quintile eating the most fiber had a 15 percent lower risk of breast cancer than did the quintile eating the least fiber. The association was strongest for postmenopausal breast cancer. A protective effect appeared for premenopausal disease, but it wasn't statistically significant.

Total dietary fiber might be associated with breast cancer protection because some of the fiber is lignan. But there's more to fiber than just lignan, and other fibers also appear protective. Once again, it all comes back to estrogen.

Beyond Lignan

When the body is finished using estrogen, it inactivates the hormone and puts it into bile. The bile is then secreted into the intestines. From there, it can be excreted from the body in stool. But bacteria in the gut make an enzyme that reactivates estrogen before it leaves the body. And this active estrogen can be reabsorbed, allowing it to once again promote breast cancer.

Fiber interferes with this bacterial enzyme. As a result, estrogen can't be reactivated or reabsorbed.[92] This unabsorbed estrogen can then be eliminated from the body with bowel movements.

If fiber keeps flushing estrogen out of the body, blood levels of estrogen should eventually drop. David Rose and coworkers from the American Health Foundation report that's exactly what happens.[93] After only two months, consumption of half an ounce of bran per day led to a significant decrease in estrogen levels.

Fiber was shown to interfere with estrogen in a Dutch report conducted at the same time as Rose's investigation. The Dutch researchers found that girls who ate more fiber from grains had lower estrogen levels as well as a delayed first menstrual cycle and delayed breast development.[94] It's probable that these delays will reduce breast cancer risk years later.

In addition to reducing breast cancer risk, fiber treats constipation. If a lack of fiber can cause constipation, then constipation should correlate with an increased risk of breast cancer. Years ago, researchers from the University of California at San Francisco found a link between constipation and precancerous changes in the breast.[95] Women with two or fewer bowel movements per week had 4.5 times the risk of precancerous breast changes than did women having a bowel movement more than once per day.

These researchers suggest that a carcinogenic substance might be lurking in stool — a substance that the body can absorb better if the stool stays in the intestine for a long time — because of constipation. Perhaps that substance is estrogen.

More Cold Water from the Nurses' Health Study

The Nurses' Health Study has investigated the link between fiber and breast cancer protection. As you might guess, the researchers did not find it, just as they couldn't find the link to dietary fat.[96] As we'll see in Chapters 13 and 14, they also didn't find selenium to be protective or obesity to be a risk factor, though most other researchers do. The Nurses' Health Study continues to report results inconsistent with those of most other research groups — which suggests that the nurses they studied were either providing inaccurate feedback about their diets or are somehow unrepresentative of most other women.

Except for the Nurses' Health Study, the animal data and human trials have been consistent. Fiber protects. Moreover, scientists have found mechanisms that explain why fiber reduces breast cancer risk, and these scientific explanations have been backed up by considerable research.

Increasing Fiber in the Diet

If you're one of the nurses from the Nurses' Health Study, you might choose to keep eating your white bread; maybe it won't make any difference. If you've decided to increase your fiber, there's good news. It's not terribly difficult.

Eat more beans and produce. Replace fruit juice with fruit, white rice with brown rice, and white bread with whole wheat bread. Some grains like oats, rye, millet, and corn don't have fiber removed when they are converted into bread, crackers, and chips. So, you don't have to look for a "whole rye" label on rye crackers; the rye is always whole. Watch out for rye bread, however; it's usually made primarily of white wheat flour.

In oriental restaurants, only white rice is available. Don't panic. The lowest breast cancer rates come from countries where white rice is eaten at every meal. But when you're at home, make brown rice. If you don't have the time, quick-cooking (15–20 minutes) brown rice is available. It doesn't taste exactly like regular brown rice, though some people actually prefer its nutty flavor.

Watch out for so-called whole wheat products. Most are a mixture of white and whole wheat flour. White flour is hidden on the ingredients list as enriched flour, unbleached flour, wheat flour, and semolina flour. Look for a label that says "100 percent whole wheat" on your loaf of bread. Supermarkets usually carry at least one brand. In health food stores, most of the wheat bread is 100 percent whole. Try as many different brands as you can. They vary considerably in taste, and you're sure to find something you like if you keep hunting. Making your own might give you the best results; electric bread makers make it a fairly easy process.

In restaurants, real whole wheat products are usually not available. Getting so-called wheat as opposed to white is often the best you can do. When restaurants refer to their baked goods as "wheat," they usually mean that a little whole wheat has been thrown in.

You won't find whole wheat pasta in restaurants, and even health food stores may carry only one brand, compared with a dozen kinds of white flour noodles. Whole wheat pasta is heavy, so many people don't like it; that's why it's hard to find on the shelves. Try it once before discarding the idea, though. Get the thinnest whole wheat noodles available. Whole wheat fettucini is easier to chew than are wide noodles. Health food stores also carry other whole-grain pastas made from brown rice, barley, spelt, amaranth, and quinoa.

If you're trying to increase your intake of lignan specifically, add flaxseed. And don't let the folks in the health food store confuse it with psyllium seed. They're not the same thing.

Your taste buds might need a period of transition when you switch to a high-fiber diet. But after you get used to the real thing, you'll find everything else bland.

ANTICANCER FOODS

From the American Cancer Society to laetrile clinics in Tijuana, Mexico, virtually everyone agrees: fruits and vegetables reduce the risk of cancer. Even the Nurses' Health Study found vegetables protective against breast cancer.[97] The Geoffrey Howe compilation of twelve studies reported higher fruit and vegetable intakes in healthy women than in breast cancer patients.[98]

Until recently, scientists assumed this protection resulted primarily from antioxidants — nutrients that prevent damage to DNA, the cellular machinery needed to reproduce cells. When DNA is damaged, cellular replication becomes abnormal and cancer is more likely to occur.* But in the last few years, researchers

---

*The common antioxidants, vitamin C, vitamin E, beta-carotene, and selenium are widely available as supplements in health food stores. Each is discussed in the next chapter. Appendix C lists foods high in these antioxidants.

have recently discovered cancer-fighting substances in produce. These natural chemicals are neither vitamins nor minerals. Most are not antioxidants nor are they even considered nutrients. But they do protect animals from cancer and are also found in the foods associated with cancer prevention in women.

Cruciferous Vegetables

Cauliflower, broccoli, cabbage, and brussels sprouts belong to the group of vegetables labeled "cruciferous." All are linked to cancer prevention. One of the chemicals found in these vegetables, indole-3-carbinol (I3C), is of special interest to breast cancer researchers because of its effect on estrogen metabolism.

Estrogen can be processed through two pathways. One of these pathways activates estrogen. The other deactivates it. When men and women are fed I3C, estrogen favors the deactivation pathway[99] and is no longer available for activation by the competing pathway.

In animal studies, I3C reduces mammary cancer.[100] Researchers in this field have high hopes that the I3C in cruciferous vegetables will also protect women from breast cancer, though other chemicals in these same vegetables also look promising.

For example, broccoli contains sulforaphane, another anticancer substance. Sulforaphane increases the activity of enzymes that detoxify cancer-causing agents. Paul Talalay, the leading sulforaphane researcher, has said it's "possibly the most potent protective agent [against cancer] yet discovered."[101] Sulforaphane is one of a group of chemicals called isothiocyanates found in all cruciferous vegetables. As a group, isothiocyanates decrease mammary cancer in animals.[102]

Foods Containing Glucaric Acid

Broccoli contains yet another anticancer substance — glucaric acid, which interferes with mammary cancer in rats.[103] Scientists believe it promotes the body's ability to excrete cancer-causing chemicals.

Although supplements containing glucaric acid are available in some health food stores, the amount used in animal research exceeds currently available supplement doses. The appropriate amount for humans to take is unknown. Foods (other than broccoli) high in glucaric acid include oranges, carrots, spinach, and apples.[104]

Soybeans

Women whose diets include an abundance of soybean products have a low risk of breast cancer.[105] Rats fed soybeans have a reduced mammary cancer risk.[106] Recently, scientists have begun to understand why soybeans protect us.

Soybeans contain genistein,* a substance that interferes with the formation of new blood vessels.[107] Tumors need an unusual amount of blood. Therefore, researchers believe soy may protect us in part by starving the tumor of its blood supply. In fact, anything that disrupts a tumor's blood supply is considered a potential anticancer agent. (See the discussion of shark cartilage in Chapter 10.) Some researchers believe genistein's anticancer effect comes partially from its ability to act as an antioxidant.[108] This multifaceted chemical also appears to protect against breast cancer by altering estrogen metabolism.

Genistein, along with equol and daidzein, two other soy-derived substances, are called phytoestrogens. Phytoestrogens are chemicals extracted from plants; scientists believe these chemicals act like tamoxifen but without the side effects.[109] Women consuming the traditional Japanese diet associated with cancer protection excrete 1,000 times more genistein than do women from societies with high breast cancer rates.[110] They also excrete high levels of equol and daidzein.

Like broccoli, soybeans contain multiple protective ingredients. Recently, some soy researchers have become interested in

---

*The other plant containing genistein, red clover, is in the Hoxsey formula discussed in Chapter 10.

Bowman-Birk protease inhibitor, another soy-derived substance that reduces cancer in animals.[111]

Tofu, miso, and soy sauce are the primary sources of all of these unique soybean protectors. Soybean dishes also make good sources, and roasted soy beans are available in health food stores.

Tomatoes — A Source of Lycopene

Lycopene is related in structure to beta-carotene, one of the common antioxidants; because of the structural similarity, it's called a carotenoid. In 1989, researchers discovered that lycopene is a more powerful antioxidant than beta-carotene or any other carotenoid.[112] Tomatoes are the best source of lycopene. Supplements containing a "mixture of carotenoids," including lycopene, are beginning to appear in some health food stores, but their lycopene content is low. The best way to increase your intake of this potent antioxidant is to eat tomatoes. Whether lycopene will protect against breast cancer has not yet been studied, though antioxidants in general have anticancer activity and lycopene is a powerful antioxidant.

ORGANICALLY GROWN FOOD

Ads in the *Washington Post, USA Today,* and the *New York Times* have boldly stated "our food supply is safe."[113] The sponsor of these ads, The American Council on Science and Health, is funded by the pesticide industry.[114]

The Politics of Pesticides

According to the Environmental Protection Agency's own data, at least sixty-seven currently used pesticides cause cancer in animals.[115] When extensively tested, almost all animal carcinogens are eventually found to cause cancer in humans.

Until recently, the issue of pesticides and cancer risks was imbued with emotion — not science. For most human cancers, a lack of hard evidence still separates pesticide exposure from clear cancer risks. With breast cancer, however, a relationship is emerging and for good reasons. Pesticide residues collect in fatty tissue, making the breast a prime reservoir for "hazardous wastes." And several pesticides, like endosulfan, currently used on grapes, lettuce, and tomatoes, have estrogenic effects.

In 1990, Finnish researchers reported that women with high levels of a pesticide (hexachlorocyclohexane) in their breasts had more than ten times the normal risk of breast cancer.[116] At the same time, researchers from Jerusalem were uncovering related clues in their attempt to understand a previously inexplicable drop in Israeli breast cancer rates.

During the decade between 1976 and 1986, breast cancer in Israel decreased almost 8 percent overall, despite a dietary increase in animal fat and alcohol and a reduction in fruit and vegetable intake. *For women under 45, breast cancer rates dropped more than 30 percent.** Researchers noted a correlation between these surprising declines and a ban (early in the decade) on the use of the pesticides hexachlorocyclohexane and lindane plus a dramatic drop in the use of DDT.[117] All three pesticides cause cancer in animals. DDT also has estrogenic effects.

In 1992, American researchers reported that breast cancer patients have ten times more DDT residue in their breasts than do other women.[118] They also found elevated levels of PCBs. Women with higher blood levels of DDT breakdown products were recently reported to have four times the normal breast cancer risk.[119] In 1994, Canadian researchers also found the relationship with a DDT breakdown product, but it was limited to women with positive estrogen-receptor status.[120] Remember that DDT has an estrogenic effect. Therefore, it makes sense that women who have more receptors for estrogen might be more affected by DDT exposure. Although DDT was banned in the United States more than twenty years ago, residues continue to show up in breast tissue.

---

*One of our editors suggested italicizing this sentence and made the following comment: "If any of those chemo studies had shown a 30 percent drop in breast cancer rates, they'd be adding it to the water supply."

Before the ban, the Food and Drug Administration (FDA) assured us DDT was safe. The FDA still asserts that all currently used pesticides are safe.[121] The FDA is able to make this claim in part by underestimating what we eat.[122] For example, the agency officially assumes each person eats one-half of one cantaloupe per year. That's it. By making this assumption, it's possible to declare that whatever toxic residue remains on that lonely half melon doesn't pose a meaningful cancer risk.

The Environmental Protection Agency (EPA) and the FDA are charged with protecting us from carcinogens in food.* During the 1980s, both agencies looked for loopholes to circumvent the law. But as a result of a decision that the Supreme Court has let stand, the National Resources Defense Council has recently forced the EPA to begin complying with the law.[123] But the National Agricultural Chemicals Association may attempt to have the law changed.

Reducing Your Pesticide Exposure

How can you take care of yourself while all this politicking is going on? The easiest way to reduce pesticide exposure is to give up animal fat. "Animal fat? They don't spray the pigs." That's true. But animals concentrate pesticide residues from their feed as well as other sources. Beef, pork, and chicken are on the National Academy of Science's list of foods posing the greatest cancer risk as a result of pesticide residues.† Freshwater fish aren't on the list but are exposed to pesticides in rivers and lakes. Replacing them with fish from the ocean will reduce pesticide exposure. Some health food stores carry frozen Icelandic fish caught in non-polluted waters.

How about organically raised meat? Cathy and I avoid it, along with commercially raised meat. Organically raised meat reduces pesticide exposure, but the level of animal fat found in such meat is not invariably lower. We simply don't know how

---

*The Delaney Clause, passed in 1958, prohibits cancer-causing chemicals in the food supply.

†The others are tomatoes, apples, lettuce, carrots, wheat, soybeans, and grapes.

much of the link between animal fat and cancer is a function of pesticide residues and how much is not.

In lieu of going strictly organic, you can reduce your pesticide exposure from produce with the following tips:

- When possible, avoid imported produce, which typically has higher pesticide residues than does domestically grown produce.
- Wash produce with soap and water to reduce (though not eliminate) exposure.
- Peel all waxed produce such as cucumbers. (Ask about apples — some species are waxed by people and others are "waxed" by nature.)
- Don't worry about bananas, corn, grapefruit, melons, and oranges. Pesticide residues tend to not penetrate their peels and husks.
- Consider buying the organically grown variety of items you eat frequently — tomatoes and lettuce, for example.

Cathy and I buy organically grown produce whenever possible. We also use organically grown tomato sauce, brown rice, oats, popcorn, and crackers. But when attempting to reduce pesticide exposure is not practical (when we're eating at someone else's house or at a restaurant), we just let it go.

But you might want to consider switching to organically grown produce. If you've never bought organically grown food before, prepare to pay a hefty price. Also, brace yourself for the worm hidden on top of each ear of corn. At first, I was appalled; now, when eating commercial corn, I realize the worm's not there because it knows better.

Regarding our organic transformation, we're frequently asked "Does it taste better?" Sometimes yes, sometimes no. But from our point of view, we're buying health insurance, not taste.

THE BIG PICTURE

Got it? It's not as complicated as the details make it seem. Eat lots of vegetables, fruit, whole grains, fish, soy products, and nonfat yogurt. Stop eating meat, fowl, eggs, fried foods, fat-containing dairy products, and junk. Cut way back on sugar. Use olive oil. See Appendix A, "Making the Transition: Eating In, Eating Out."

References

1. Willett, W. C., et al. Dietary fat and fiber in relation to risk of breast cancer. *JAMA* 1992;268:2037–44.

2. Prentiss, R. Breast cancer from diet, tobacco, and alcohol. *JAMA* 1993;269:1790–1 [letter].

3. Wynder, E. L., L. Cohen, and S. D. Stellman. Letter. *JAMA* 1993;269:1791.

4. Cohen, M. H. Letter. *JAMA* 1993;269:1791.

5. Boyd, N. F., et al. Dietary fat and breast cancer risk: the feasibility of a clinical trial of breast cancer prevention. *Lipids* 1992;27:821–6.

6. Fackelmann, K. A. Dietary fat: no link to breast cancer. *Sci News* 1993; 142:276.

7. Raloff, J. EcoCancers—do environmental factors underlie a breast cancer epidemic? *Sci News* 1993;144:10–13.

8. Carroll, K. K., et al. Dietary fat and mammary cancer. *Can Med Assoc J* 1968;98:590–3.

9. Goodwin, P. J., and N. F. Boyd. Critical appraisal of the evidence that dietary fat intake is related to breast cancer risk in humans. *J Natl Cancer Inst* 1987;79:473–85 [review].

10. Freedman, L. S., C. Clifford, and M. Messina. Analysis of dietary fat, calories, body weight, and the development of mammary tumors in rats and mice: a review. *Cancer Res* 1990;50:5710–9.

11. Tannenbaum, A. The genesis and growth of tumors. III. Effects of a high-fat diet. *Cancer Res* 1942;2:468–75.

12. Merzenich, H., H. Boeing, and J. Wahrendorf. Dietary fat and sports activity as determinants for age at menarche. *Am J Epidemiol* 1993;138:217–24.

13. Goldin, B. R., et al. The relationship between estrogen levels and diets of Caucasian American and Oriental immigrant women. *Am J Clin Nutr* 1986;44:945–53.

14. Prentice, R., et al. Dietary fat reduction and plasma estradiol concentration of healthy postmenopausal women. *J Natl Cancer Inst* 1990;82:129–34.

15. McDougall, J. A. Preliminary study of diet as an adjunct therapy for breast cancer. *Breast* 1984;10:18–21.

16. Goodwin, P. J., and N. F. Boyd. Critical appraisal of the evidence that dietary fat intake is related to breast cancer risk in humans. *J Natl Cancer Inst* 1987;79:473–85 [review].

17. Henderson, M. M. International differences in diet and cancer incidence. *J Natl Cancer Inst Monogr* 1992;12:59–63.

18. Wynder, E. L., et al. A comparison of survival rates between American and Japanese patients with breast cancer. *Surg Gynecol Obstet* 1963;117:196–200.

19. Sakamoto, G., H. Sugano, and W. H. Hartmann. Comparative clinicopathological study of breast cancer among Japanese and American females. *Jpn J Cancer Clin* 1979;25:161–70.

20. Haenszel, W., and M. Kurihara. Studies of Japanese migrants. I. Mortality from cancer and other diseases among Japanese in the United States. *J Natl Cancer Inst* 1968;40:43–68.

21. Shimizu, H., et al. Cancer of the prostate and breast among Japanese and white immigrants of Los Angeles county. *Br J Cancer* 1991;63:963–6.

22. Ziegler R. G., et al. Migration patterns and breast cancer risk in Asian-American women. *J Natl Cancer Inst* 1993;85:1819–27.

23. Wynder, E. L., and L. A. Cohen. A rationale for dietary intervention in the treatment of postmenopausal breast cancer patients. *Nutr Cancer* 1982;3:195–9.

24. Holm, L-E., et al. Treatment failure and dietary habits in women with breast cancer. *J Natl Cancer Inst* 1993;85:32–6.

25. Nomura, A. M. Y., et al. The effect of dietary fat on breast cancer survival among Caucasian and Japanese women in Hawaii. *Breast Cancer Res Treatment* 1991;18:S135–41.

26. McDougall, J. A. Preliminary study of diet as adjunct therapy for breast cancer. *Breast* 1984;10:18–21.

27. Boyd, N. F., et al. Dietary fat and breast cancer risk: the feasibility of a clinical trial of breast cancer prevention. *Lipids* 1992;27:821–6.

28. Boyar, A. P., et al. Response to a diet low in total fat in women with postmenopausal breast cancer: a pilot study. *Nutr Cancer* 1988;11:93–9.

29. Longcope, C., et al. The effect of a low fat diet on estrogen metabolism. *J Clin Endocrinol Metabol* 1987;64:1246–50.

30. Goodwin, P. J., and N. F. Boyd. Critical appraisal of the evidence that dietary fat intake is related to breast cancer risk in humans. *J Natl Cancer Inst* 1987;79:473–85.

31. Toniolo, P., et al. Calorie-providing nutrients and risk of breast cancer. *J Natl Cancer Inst* 1989;81:278–86.

32. Rohan, T. E., A. J. McMichael, and P. A. Bagjusrt. A population-based case-control study of diet and breast cancer in Australia. *Am J Epidemiol* 1988;128:478–89.

33. Howe, G. R., et al. Dietary factors and risk of breast cancer: combined analysis of 12 case-control studies. *J Natl Cancer Inst* 1990;82:561–9.

34. Katsouyanni, K. et al. Diet and breast cancer: a case-control study in Greece. *Int J Cancer* 1986;38:815–20.

35. Howe, G. R. High-fat diets and breast cancer risk—the epidemiologic evidence. *JAMA* 1992;268:2080–1 [editorial].

36. Howe, G. R., et al. A cohort study of fat intake and risk of breast cancer. *J Natl Cancer Inst* 1991;83:336–40.

37. van den Brandt, P. A., et al. A prospective cohort study on dietary fat and the risk of postmenopausal breast cancer. *Cancer Res* 1993;53:75–82.

38. Kushi, L. H., et al. Dietary fat and postmenopausal breast cancer. *J Natl Cancer Inst* 1992;84:1092–9.

39. Graham, S., et al. Diet in the epidemiology of postmenopausal breast cancer in the New York state cohort. *Am J Epidemiol* 1992;136:1327–37.

40. Barrett-Connor, E., and N. J. Friedlander. Dietary fat, calories, and the risk of breast cancer in postmenopausal women: a prospective population-based study. *J Am Coll Nutr* 1993;12:390–9.

41. Pariza, M. W. Calories and energy expenditure in carcinogenesis. *Contemporary Nutr* 1986;XI:1–2 [review].

42. Pariza, M. W. Dietary fat, calorie restriction, ad libitum feeding, and cancer risk. *Nutr Rev* 1987;45:1–7 [review].

43. Heber, D., et al. Weight reduction for breast cancer prevention by restriction of dietary fat and calories: rationale, mechanisms and interventions. *Nutr* 1989;5:149–54 [review].

44. Tannenbaum, A. The dependence of tumor formation on the composition of the calorie-restricted diet as well as on the degree of restriction. *Cancer Res* 1945;5:616–25.

45. Boring, C. C., T. S. Squires, and T. Tong. Cancer statistics, 1993. *CA* 1993; 43:7–26.

46. Sasaki, S., M. Horacsek, and H. Kesteloot. An ecological study of the relationship between dietary fat intake and breast cancer mortality. *Prev Med* 1993;22:187–202.

47. Pritchard, G. A., D. L. Jones, and R. E. Mansel. Lipids in breast carcinogenesis. *Br J Surg* 1989;76:1069–73.

48. Borgeson, C. E., et al. Effects of dietary fish oil on human mammary carcinoma and on lipid-metabolizing enzymes. *Lipids* 1989;24:290–5.

49. Kaizer, L., et al. Fish consumption and breast cancer risk: an ecological study. *Nutr Cancer* 1989;12:61–8.

50. Baxevanis, C. N., et al. Elevated prostaglandin E2 production by monocytes is responsible for the depressed levels of natural killer and lymphokine-activated killer cell function in patients with breast cancer. *Cancer* 1993;72:491–501.

51. Cohen, L. A., et al. Dietary fat and mammary cancer. 1. Promoting effects of different dietary fats on *n*-nitrosomethylurea-induced rat mammary tumorigenesis. *J Natl Cancer Inst* 1986;77:33–42.

52. Tinsley, I. J., J. A. Schmitz, and D. A. Pierce. Influence of dietary fatty acids on the incidence of mammary tumors in the C3H mouse. *Cancer Res* 1981;41:1460–5.

53. Reddy, B. S., and Y. Maeura. Tumor promotion by dietary fat in azoxymethan-induced colon carcinogenesis in female F344 rats: influence of amount and source of dietary fat. *J Natl Cancer Inst* 1984;72:745–50.

54. Perez, R. V., et al. Altered macrophage function in dietary immunoregulation. *J Parenteral Enteral Nutr* 1989;13:1–10.

55. Wynder, E. L., et al. Diet and breast cancer in causation and therapy. *Cancer* 1984;58:1804–13 [review].

56. Keys, A., et al. The diet and 15-year death rate in the seven countries study. *Am J Epidemiol* 1986;124:903–15.

57. Shun-Zhang Y, et al. A case-control study of dietary and nondietary risk factors for breast cancer in Shanghai. *Cancer Res* 1990;50:5017–21.

58. Sasaki, S., M. Moracsek, and H. Kesteloot. An ecological study of the relationship between dietary fat intake and breast cancer mortality. *Prev Med* 1993;22:187–202.

59. Verreault, R., et al. Dietary fat in relation to prognostic indicators in breast cancer. *J Natl Cancer Inst* 1988;80:819–25.

60. Ingram, D. M., E. M. Nottage, and A. N. Roberts. Prolactin and breast cancer risk. *Med J Austr* 1990;153:469–73.

61. Hirayama, T. Life-style and cancer: from epidemiological evidence to public behavior change to mortality reduction of target cancers. *J Natl Cancer Inst Monogr* 1992;12:65–74.

62. La Vecchia, C., and S. Pampallona. Age at first birth, dietary practices and breast cancer mortality in various Italian regions. *Oncology* 1986;43:1–6.

63. Drasar, B. S., and D. Irving. Environmental factors and cancer of the colon and breast. *Br J Cancer* 1973;27:167–72 [review].

64. Richardson, S., M. Gerber, and S. Cenée. The role of fat, animal protein and some vitamin consumption in breast cancer: a case control study in southern France. *Int J Cancer* 1991;48:1–9.

65. Willett, W. C., et al. Intake of *trans* fatty acids and risk of coronary heart disease among women. *Lancet* 1993;341:581–5.

66. Awad, A. B. Trans fatty acids in tumor development and the host survival. *J Natl Cancer Inst* 1981;67:189–92.

67. Drasar, B. S., and D. Irving. Environmental factors and cancer of the colon and breast. *Br J Cancer* 1973;27:167–72 [review].

68. Lee, H. P., et al. Dietary effects on breast-cancer risk in Singapore. *Lancet* 1991;337:1197–2000.

69. Lubin, F., Y. Wax, and B. Modan. Role of fat, animal protein, and dietary fiber in breast cancer etiology: a case-control study. *J Natl Cancer Inst* 1986;77:605–12

70. Van't Veer, P., et al. Combination of dietary factors in relation to breast cancer occurrence. *Int J Cancer* 1991;47:649–53.

71. Lê M. G., et al. Consumption of dairy produce and alcohol in a case-control study of breast cancer. *J Natl Cancer Inst* 1986;77:633–6.

72. Curhan, G. C., et al. A prospective study of dietary calcium and other nutrients and the risk of symptomatic kidney stones. *N Engl J Med* 1993;328:833–8.

73. Lea, A. J. Dietary factors associated with death-rates from certain neoplasms in man. *Lancet* 1966;ii:332–3.

74. Hankin, J. H., P. H. Rawlings, and V. Rawlings. Diet and breast cancer: a review. *Am J Clin Nutr* 1978;31:2005.

75. Kalamegham, R., and K. K. Carrol. Reversal of the promotional effect of high-fat diet on mammary tumorigenesis by subsequent lowering of dietary fat. *Nutr Cancer* 1984;6:22.

76. Kushi, L. H., et al. Dietary fat and postmenopausal breast cancer. *J Natl Cancer Inst* 1992;84:1092.

77. Sasaki, S., M. Horacsek, and H. Kesteloot. An ecological study of the relationship between dietary fat intake and breast cancer mortality. *Prev Med* 1993;22:187–202.

78. Verreault, R., et al. Dietary fat in relation to prognostic indicators in breast cancer. *J Natl Cancer Inst* 1988;80:819–25.

79. Lee, H. P., et al. Dietary effects on breast-cancer risk in Singapore. *Lancet* 1991;337:1197–2000.

80. Walker, B. E. Tumors in female offspring of control and diethylstilbestrol-exposed mice fed high-fat diets. *J Natl Cancer Inst* 1990;82:50–4.

81. Raloff, J. Mom's fatty diet may induce child's cancer. *Sci News* 1990;137:5.

82. Rennie, S. Breast cancer prevention: diet vs. drugs. *Ms.* 1993;III:38–45.

83. Cohen, L. A., D. P. Rose, and E. L. Wynder. A rationale for dietary intervention in postmenopausal breast cancer patients: an update. *Nutr Cancer* 1993;19:1–10.

84. Carroll, K. K. Dietary fat and breast cancer. *Lipids* 1992;27:793–7 [review].

85. Boyd, N. F., et al. Dietary fat and breast cancer risk: the feasibility of a clinical trial of breast cancer prevention. *Lipids* 1992;27:821–6.

86. Adlercreutz, H. Does fiber-rich food containing animal lignan precursors protect against both colon and breast cancer: an extension of the fiber hypothesis. *Gastroenterol* 1984;86:761–6 [editorial/review].

87. Adlercreutz, H., et al. Excretion of the lignans enterolactone and enterodiol and of equol in omnivorous and vegetarian postmenopausal women and in women with breast cancer. *Lancet* 1982;ii:1295–9.

88. Adlercreutz, H., et al. Determination of urinary lignans and phytoestrogen metabolites, potential antiestrogens and anticarcinogens, in urine of women on various habitual diets. *J Steroid Biochem* 1986;25:791–7.

89. Carroll, K. K., and T. T. Khor. Effects of level and type of dietary fat on incidence of mammary tumors induced in female sprague-dawley rats by dimethylbenz[a]anthracene. *Lipids* 1971;6:415–20.

90. van't Veer, P., et al. Dietary fiber, beta-carotene and breast cancer: results from a case-control study. *Int J Cancer* 1990;45:825–8.

91. Howe, G. R., et al. Dietary factors and risk of breast cancer: combined analysis of 12 case-control studies. *J Natl Cancer Inst* 1990;82:561–9.

92. Rose, D. P. Dietary fiber and breast cancer. *Nutr Cancer* 1990;13:1–8 [review].

93. Rose, D. P., et al. High-fiber diet reduces serum estrogen concentrations in premenopausal women. *Am J Clin Nutr* 1991;54:520–5.

94. de Ridder, C. M., et al. Dietary habits, sexual maturation, and plasma hormones in pubertal girls: a longitudinal study. *Am J Clin Nutr* 1991;54:805–13.

95. Petrakis, N. L., and E. B. King. Cytological abnormalities in nipple aspirates of breast fluid from women with severe constipation. *Lancet* 1981;ii:1203–5.

96. Willett, W. C., et al. Dietary fat and fiber in relation to risk of breast cancer. *JAMA* 1992;268:2037–44.

97. Hunter, D. J., et al. A prospective study of the intake of vitamins C, E, and the risk of breast cancer. *N Engl J Med* 1993;329:234–40.

98. Howe, G. R., et al. Dietary factors and risk of breast cancer: combined analysis of 12 case-control studies. *J Natl Cancer Inst* 1990;82:561–9.

99. Michnovicz, J. J., and H. L. Bradlow. Altered estrogen metabolism and excretion in humans following consumption of indole-3-carbinol. *Nutr Cancer* 1991;16:59–66.

100. Wattenberg, L. W., and W. D. Loub. Inhibition of polycyclic aromatic hydrocarbon-induced neoplasia by naturally occurring indoles. *Cancer Res* 1978;38:1410–13.

101. Stroh, M. Inside broccoli: a weapon against cancer. *Sci News* 1992;141:183.

102. Wattenberg, L. W. Inhibition of carcinogenesis by minor anutrient constituents of the diet. *Proc Nutri Soc* 1990;49:173–83 [review].

103. Abou-Issa, H. M., et al. Putative metabolites derived from dietary combinations of calcium glucarate and N-(4-hydroxyphenyl) retinamide act synergistically to inhibit the induction of rat mammary tumors by 7,12–dimethylbenz[a]anthracene. *Proc Natl Acad Sci* 1988;85;4181–4.

104. Dwivedi, C., et al. Effect of calcium glucarate on β-glucuronidase activity

and glucarate content of certain vegetables and fruits. *Biochem Med Metabol Biol* 1990;43:83–92.

105. Lee, H. P., et al. Dietary effects on breast-cancer risk in Singapore. *Lancet* 1991;337:1197–1200.

106. Barnes, S. Anti-cancer substances in soybeans—potential involvement in breast cancer. American Cancer Society's Thirty-second Science Writers Seminar, Daytona Beach, Florida, March 27, 1990.

107. Fotsis, T., et al. Genistein, a dietary-derived inhibitor of *in vitro* angiogenesis. *Proc Natl Acad Sci* 1993;90:2690–4.

108. Wei, H., et al. Inhibition of tumor promoter-induced hydrogen peroxide formation *in vitro* and *in vivo* by genistein. *Nutr Cancer* 1993;20:1–12.

109. Fackelmann, K. A. Blocking breast cancer. *Sci News* 1990;137:296–7.

110. Adlercreutz, H., et al. Dietary phyto-oestrogens and the menopause in Japan. *Lancet* 1992;339:1233 [letter].

111. Messina, M., and S. Barnes. The role of soy products in reducing risk of cancer. *J Natl Cancer Inst* 1991;83:541–6 [review].

112. DiMascio, P., S. Kaiser, and H. Sies. Lycopene as the most efficient biological carotenoid singlet oxygen quencher. *Arch Biochem Biophys* 1989;274;532–8.

113. American Council on Science and Health. Advertisement, *USA Today*, April 5, 1989, p. 9A.

114. Lefferts, L. Y. Pesticides: facts vs. fantasy. *Nutrition Action* 1989;16(5):8–9.

115. Corliss, J. The Delaney Clause: too much of a good thing? *J Natl Cancer Inst* 1993;85:600–3.

116. Mussalo-Rauhamaa, H., et al. Occurrence of beta-hexachlorocyclohexane in breast cancer patients. *Cancer* 1990;66:2124–28.

117. Westin, J. B., and E. Richter. The Israeli breast-cancer anomaly. *Ann NY Acad Sci* 1990;609:269–79.

118. Falck, F., et al. Pesticides and polychlorinated biphenyl residues in human breast lipids and their relation to breast cancer. *Arch Environ Health* 1992;47:143–6.

119. Wolff, M. S., et al. Blood levels of organochlorine residues and risk of breast cancer. *J Natl Cancer Inst* 1993;85:648–52.

120. Dewailly E., et al. High organochlorine body burden in women with estrogen receptor-positive breast cancer. *J Natl Cancer Inst* 1994;86:232–4.

121. Wessel, J. R. The extent of pesticide residues in the food supply. *J Assoc Food Drug Officials* 1988;52(A):52–6.

122. Montgomery, A. America's pesticide-permeated food. *Nutrition Action* 1987; 14(5):1,4–7.

123. Corliss, J. The Delaney Clause: too much of a good thing? *J Natl Cancer Inst* 1993;85:600–3.

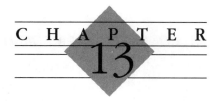

CHAPTER 13

Supplements and
Prevention

STEVE

*"Today many [conventional] physicians admit that complementary
medicine has some potential and deserves a fair trial. Thus the
anxiety of the profession is growing."*[1]

Edzard Ernst, Professor of Medicine,
Hanover Medical School, Germany

Your medical doctor is likely to tell you there is no proof that taking supplements can reduce your risk of breast cancer or a recurrence. At the moment, this is technically true, though several
studies in progress will assess whether certain supplements play a
role in cancer prevention.

Statements about lack of proof are often followed by another comment, usually said with an air of condescension: "You
can take vitamins if you want; they probably won't hurt." There's
an unstated implication here: Anything that won't hurt you can't
be "strong" enough to do you any good. But, remember, you're
not fighting a nuclear war. You're trying to heal.

Results of studies on the ability of supplements to reduce
cancer risk will not be available for years. Even then, these initial
studies will probably not be totally conclusive. Yet there are valid
scientific reasons to consider using several supplements, despite
the current lack of absolute proof.

SUPPLEMENTS AND CONVENTIONAL MEDICAL PHILOSOPHY

Many medical doctors tend to make the philosophical mistake of unconsciously assuming that if something is not proven, it doesn't work. Consciously, we can all understand the fallacy of this position. It's tantamount to suggesting that before the link between vitamin C deficiency and scurvy was proven, people who ate foods rich in vitamin C were no better off than sailors on hardtack. A school child can see beyond this line of reasoning. But when such an assumption is made unconsciously, it can cloud the minds of remarkably intelligent people.

In fact, in 1753, when James Lind published his treatise on the relationship between foods containing vitamin C and protection against scurvy, the medical establishment considered his work insufficient proof. English sailors continued to die until the medical profession finally conceded forty years later.

As a result of the "if it's not proven, it can't work" philosophy, numerous effective treatments and preventive agents have been and are currently being ignored by many conventional medical doctors. Scientists refer to the mistake made when a useful intervention is considered useless because of lack of absolute proof as a "type II error."

Conventional medical doctors make many type II errors, but not without good reason. If you deal with dangerous substances, you must be sure that these therapies do something useful before prescribing them to patients. The implementation of a therapy may be postponed by a few years while it's being proven. Although some precious time is lost in the process, the alternative — employing dangerous treatments, some of which turn out to be useless — could be a disaster. Thus, to avoid Thalidomide-like catastrophes, medical doctors are willing to make some type II errors, and they should be.

But this kind of thinking doesn't make the same sense when we're talking about vitamin C. It's not chemotherapy. If a substance is inexpensive, has been proven safe, and reduces the risk of cancer in animals, should you really wait ten years for proof to develop before taking it, especially when you may not have ten years to wait?

What if we're wrong, and the vitamin eventually proves useless? Then we have made what's called a "type I error." This happens whenever a therapy is incorrectly labeled useful on the basis of what ultimately turns out to have been insufficient evidence. With vitamin C, it's unlikely that many tragedies are in the making if we commit a type I error. It's rarely toxic. All you lose is the cost of the pills.

Several supplements have been shown to be safe and also able to reduce cancer risks in animals. Moreover, these same substances have been linked with known mechanisms that explain *why* they prevent cancer. And epidemiological studies have shown that people who eat more and/or have higher blood levels of these substances have a lower susceptibility to cancer. Getting interested? You should be. (If your medical doctor finds this topic of academic interest only, it's probably because your medical doctor does not have breast cancer.)

Why are many medical doctors turned off by the debate over supplements? I've encountered a surprising level of emotional reactivity when I challenge the medical establishment's handling of type I and type II errors with respect to supplements. Many conventional medical doctors have confused their opinions with science; perhaps they don't want to be reminded that choosing to lean toward type II errors is not a scientific choice. It's a human choice, a subjective choice, a choice that makes sense with dangerous drugs but not with harmless substances. But the discomfort shown by conventional doctors when these topics are posed ultimately goes beyond that.

Part of the explanation lies in the fact that medical doctors receive very little training in nutrition. The Center for Science in the Public Interest tells us that only 24 percent of medical schools require a nutrition course and 60 percent provide fewer than 20 hours of nutrition education.[2] Some of this lack of education is now being corrected by adding a basic course, albeit with limited hours. A large body of scientific evidence shows the clinical efficacy of food and supplements, but this information is not taught in these introductory nutrition classes. So clinical nutrition is usually foreign to medical doctors. And most people have a built-in resistance to what they know little about.

Don't be intimidated if your medical doctors' discomfort masquerades as condescension. By the time you've read this chapter, you may know much more about supplements and cancer prevention than they do.

PRIMARY PREVENTION, SECONDARY PREVENTION

You may be reading this chapter to reduce your or your daughter's risk of ever getting breast cancer. Strategies designed for this purpose are called "primary prevention." As we'll see, there are reasons to expect that supplements can contribute to primary prevention.

You may already have a breast cancer diagnosis. If you've had your initial treatments and are currently disease-free, you are now focusing on preventing a recurrence. This is called "secondary prevention." While little is known about the role supplements play in secondary prevention of breast cancer, it makes good sense to follow the same path as the healthy woman seeking primary prevention. This approach has proven to be true for most diseases and is most likely to prove true in the future for breast cancer as well. Let's look at some examples of how primary and secondary prevention strategies overlap in regard to other diseases.

We all know a person can reduce her risk of heart attack by exercise and avoidance of smoking, dietary cholesterol, and saturated fat. These same strategies are used to treat patients who have already had a heart attack. In other words, the primary prevention tools can be used to achieve secondary prevention.

Exercise and calcium supplements are part of the primary prevention of osteoporosis. Both are also used when someone has suffered an osteoporosis-related fracture, as a way to prevent a second occurrence.

People who drink a lot of water are at lower risk of getting kidney stones than are those who don't. When a patient has had a kidney stone, the doctor's first instruction to prevent a second stone is often "drink more water."

Avoiding sunburn can reduce the risk of skin cancer. Once a skin cancer has been removed, the first instruction a patient is usually given is to avoid too much sun.

This pattern of overlap between primary and secondary prevention is the rule, not the exception. I stress it here because, as we shall see, there are relatively clear reasons for using certain supplements to achieve some level of primary prevention. But technically speaking, we know almost nothing about supplements and secondary prevention of breast cancer. Therefore, we have to make the reasonable assumption that, as with other diseases, primary prevention strategies work for secondary prevention as well.

Our only current piece of evidence that primary and secondary breast cancer prevention are linked comes from Japan. Here, primary prevention (probably a function of diet) has been linked with low breast cancer risk. But when a woman in Japan does get breast cancer, her chance of never having a recurrence is known to be significantly better than that of her American counterpart. The only plausible reason appears to be the obvious: She continues to do the things that reduced her risk of breast cancer in the first place.

Before leaving this topic, we must distinguish secondary prevention from treatment. Several aspects of the Gerson therapy discussed in Chapter 10 constitute the ultimate lifestyle for achieving low cancer risk. Yet the late-stage patients I followed who were using this therapy did not survive. I have seen many cancer patients with active disease who tried to use nutritional supplements for the purpose of treatment. Such an approach usually fails. It's like deciding to quit smoking to treat lung cancer.

If you're reading this book you may be a cancer patient who has already had surgery. You may find yourself disease-free (though possibly still suffering side effects from conventional treatments). Remember that most early-stage breast cancer patients remain disease-free for many years. If you are disease-free and are trying to prevent a recurrence (secondary prevention), taking those supplements that appear to be linked with primary prevention makes sense.

ANTIOXIDANTS AND PREVENTION

The cells in your body are made of tiny units called molecules. The chemical symbol H_2O represents a molecule of water — the absolute smallest amount of water that's still water. Molecules, in turn, are made of atoms. For example, the "O" in H_2O represents an atom of oxygen. Each atom is made of still smaller parts. One of these smaller parts, the electron, likes company.

Electrons hang out in pairs. They have a phobia about spending time alone. When an electron isn't coupled up with a mate, it will work hard to rectify the situation. And it won't always wait for a matchmaker or a dating agency. It will steal another electron from some other part of your body. But this now leaves some other electron suddenly without its mate, and it too will break up yet another happy marriage of electrons. This chain reaction can cause damage, much of which is initially triggered by oxygen.

Your body needs oxygen. But oxygen does things that increase the number of lonely and dangerous electrons — a situation leading to what is called oxidative damage. Other substances can also produce unpaired electrons, and the resulting damage is collectively called "free radical pathology."

Free radicals are substances that contain unpaired electrons. They can even damage DNA — the part of each cell needed for cellular reproduction. When DNA is damaged, abnormal cells are produced. Free radical damage to DNA has been directly linked with breast cancer.[3]

An antioxidant is a substance that acts like a dating agency. It can provide a single electron as a match for a lonely unpaired electron. Once the antioxidant donates an electron, it breaks the chain reaction of damage. Then, the body can go about trying to repair whatever injury was done during the electron-swapping orgy.

The most common and safe dietary antioxidants are vitamins C and E, the mineral selenium, and beta-carotene (the nontoxic vegetable form of vitamin A). Numerous studies have found that dietary intake or blood levels of one or more of these nutrients correlate inversely with overall cancer risk. Put simply, the higher the nutrient level in the diet or blood, the lower the risk of cancer.

THE FDA VERSUS SCIENCE

Despite this wealth of evidence, the Food and Drug Administration (FDA) has prevented the food and supplement industries from claiming that antioxidants protect against cancer. In reality, the inverse link between antioxidants and cancer risk has become so scientifically unequivocal that sixteen leading nutrition researchers from all over the United States have publicly attacked the FDA's decision. Writing in the conservative, peer-reviewed journal *Nutrition Reviews,* these researchers say "an incorrect conclusion has been reached to disallow a claim that antioxidant nutrients may decrease the risk of cancer. . . . [We] believe the data clearly support approval of a health claim."[4]

These scientists go on to say that regarding certain cancers (lung, stomach, esophagus, and mouth) the research data are already *"overwhelmingly consistent* [italics theirs] in showing statistically significant protective effect of higher dietary intakes of antioxidant nutrients."

The data in question come from a slew of animal studies and epidemiological studies — reports that compare cancer rates and diet from one country to the next. The FDA denys the overwhelming scientific evidence by suggesting that other possible explanations might exist that account for the cancer prevention caused by eating fruits and vegetables (the primary sources of these antioxidants).

Certainly, there are other anticancer agents in some of these foods (see Chapter 12). Nonetheless, the *Nutrition Reviews* article builds an incontrovertible argument which tears apart the FDA opinion that a health claim should not yet be made for antioxidants. The reason is simple — there is so much evidence now linking these antioxidants with prevention, and such a remarkably high percentage of the studies lean in the same direction, regardless of how these studies are done or by whom.

For years, the FDA has had a running battle with the supplement industry; for political reasons, though, the agency officially denies this. The FDA hasn't condemned hamburgers, sausage, and junk food, yet spends tax dollars on publications, such as "Myths of Vitamins," that condemn harmless supplements.[5]

Some supplement industry personnel privately believe the FDA is bullying a 90-pound weakling because drug companies are often too powerful for the agency to control. Presumably the agency needs to dominate someone. Other people believe that because the FDA is typically headed by conventional medical doctors, it views supplements as a form of competition, especially at a time when the health care reform movement is starting to expose the damage to the U.S. economy caused by the high costs of conventional medicine.

There is no way to properly assess these points of view. Nonetheless, for whatever reasons, the FDA has clearly (and even literally) been gunning for the supplement industry.

When the FDA, with guns drawn, recently broke into the Kent, Washington, office of the nutrition-oriented medical doctor Jonathan Wright, some Seattle residents were so fed up they organized protest rallies. Dr. Wright's crime was using B vitamins without preservatives (a form commonly and legally found in Europe). The FDA never explained why it needed drawn weapons to search the doctor's office.

A notable example of more standard FDA technique occurred in 1990 with the supplement tryptophan, which was linked with eosinophilia myalgia syndrome because of a manufacturing contaminant (not the tryptophan itself). Once the contaminant was isolated[6] and traced to batches from one Japanese manufacturer,[7] the Japanese government declared (uncontaminated) tryptophan safe and put it back on the market, where it can be found today. The new, purified tryptophan is not causing health problems in Japan. But the FDA, trying to obfuscate the difference between contaminated and uncontaminated tryptophan,[8] is using the affair as a ruse to push for the removal of all similar products (amino acids) from the marketplace.

Were the FDA to admit that antioxidants protect against cancer, as scientists have asked them to do, they would be perilously close to conceding that people should take supplements. If they made that acknowledgment, they would have more difficulty continuing to justify their war against the supplement industry — a war that is interfering with preventive medicine in other areas besides cancer. For instance, by 1992 virtually all scientists and doctors outside the FDA *including other U.S. governmental agencies,* like the Centers for Disease Control and Prevention in Atlanta,[9] had acknowledged that folic acid supplements prevent certain birth defects. The FDA refused to acknowledge the folic acid–birth defects relationship until late 1993, when inaction on this matter was causing a loss in credibility for the agency. In other words, the FDA had painted supplements in such a bad light that any acknowledgment of efficacy (other than treatment of deficiency diseases) would make the FDA itself look bad.

Thus the FDA seems to be resisting acknowledging the widely accepted link between antioxidants and cancer prevention so that it can maintain its own political agenda. To counter this apparent travesty of justice, troops both from the political right — Republican Senator Orrin Hatch — and the political left — Democratic Congressman Bill Richardson — have joined forces to sponsor a bill to allow the supplement industry to limit the FDA's authority over supplements. Cosponsors include Republican Senator Strom Thurmond and Democratic Congresswoman Eleanor Holmes Norton. A friend jokingly told me the last time these two people cosigned the same legislation involved the decision to fight the Civil War — "they both apparently said 'yes,' albeit on different sides." Despite this support, passage of the Hatch-Richardson bill remains in doubt. But had the FDA not repeatedly acted in indefensible ways in its dealings with the supplement industry, such a bill would never have been written. By the time you're reading this, the outcome, proposed by these strange political bedfellows, may be history.

Years ago, the FDA tried to limit over-the-counter access to supplements. American consumers were saved in 1976 by legislation sponsored by Senator William Proxmire. The agency is again proposing that vitamins be classified as drugs if dosages exceed the low levels found in the Recommended Daily Allowances.[10] If the FDA is allowed to reclassify vitamins, you won't be able to take the supplements mentioned in this chapter. They will either be outlawed, or the dose per pill will be reduced to the point where it will become impractical to take the amount you need.

VITAMIN C AND PREVENTION

When the results of twelve breast cancer/nutrition studies were pooled together, women consuming the most vitamin C were found to have a 16 percent reduction in risk of premenopausal and a 37 percent reduction in risk of postmenopausal breast cancer.[11] At least some of this protective association is the result of other anticancer substances found in fruits and vegetables — the foods high in vitamin C. Nonetheless, the evidence suggests that vitamin C may have its own protective effect. We should take the results of this study seriously because it combines the outcomes of so much research and because the relationship between vitamin C and cancer was relatively "dose dependent." This means the more vitamin C in a woman's diet, the lower her risk of breast cancer. Of the twelve studies considered, ten looked specifically at the vitamin C–breast cancer link. Nine of the ten found that high vitamin C was associated with protection. A more recent report found a link between fruit — the best dietary source of vitamin C — and breast cancer protection.[12]

As you might expect from the discussion in Chapter 12, the Nurses' Health Study could not find a link between vitamin C in food or supplements and breast cancer prevention.[13] Several other studies have also reported no protective effect.[14] Because the Nurses' Health Study used a stronger research design than the positive studies cited in the previous paragraph, it must be considered seriously.*

It's likely that the Nurses' Health Study has proven that supplemental vitamin C won't dramatically reduce risk. However, as large as the study was (1,439 breast cancer cases developed in eight years among almost 90,000 women), it still did not rule out the possibility that vitamin C reduces breast cancer risk by 5 or 10 percent.

---

*The Nurses' Health Study was a "prospective" report — meaning that women were investigated *before* they had breast cancer. Such a design eliminates some of the problems found in weaker ("retrospective") studies that depend more on the memory of participants. Retrospective studies are also flavored by the effects of the participants' knowledge that they have breast cancer when they answer the questions presented by the researcher.

Despite the Nurses' Health Study, I believe the weight of available evidence suggests that people wanting to reduce their risk of breast cancer should consider supplementing vitamin C. A recent review of the research concluded there was "strong evidence" linking vitamin C with breast cancer prevention.[15]

How Much Vitamin C Is Enough?

Although you can increase consumption of vitamin C by eating more fruits and vegetables, the levels found in supplements — thousands of milligrams — simply cannot be obtained from a good diet. While most animals manufacture the equivalent of several thousand milligrams of vitamin C per day (adjusted to human body weight), the only way humans can get this much is through supplementation. Science doesn't yet have an answer as to how much people should take.

I take 1,000 mg per day to reduce my risk of a variety of cancers. Cathy takes 12,000 mg and Linus Pauling takes 18,000 mg.

Can Vitamin C Be Toxic?

For people with diseases involving an overload of iron (such as hemachromatosis and hemosiderosis), high doses of vitamin C can be dangerous. But for most people, this isn't a problem. (Cases of vitamin-C-induced damage in iron-overloaded people are remarkably uncommon given that millions of people are taking high doses of this vitamin.) A simple lab test (serum ferritin) can rule out excessive accumulation of iron.

For some people, 10,000 mg can cause diarrhea. This condition is not serious; the mechanism causing the diarrhea is exactly the same as that for diarrhea induced by drinking too much apple juice. However, while you have diarrhea, you can't properly absorb the vitamin C. If diarrhea becomes a side effect, it is necessary to lower the dose.

Other possible problems exist with large doses of vitamin C. A few researchers have suggested that kidney stone risks might increase for rare individuals. And chewable vitamin C, like anything else that contains sugar and acid, causes tooth decay. (Most common supplement sources of vitamin C are in an acid form; these include many chewables.) Even so, this list of possible toxicities doesn't look nearly as dangerous as the list for Cytoxan (see Chapter 7). For the vast majority of people, large doses are safe. Except for the diarrhea and tooth decay from the chewables, I haven't actually seen any toxicity in anyone at any dose. But remember — anything can become toxic at some dose. Even too much water can cause a problem: It's called drowning. If you have questions, find a naturopathic (or other nutrition-oriented) physician.

BETA-CAROTENE AND PREVENTION

Another valuable anticancer supplement is vitamin A, which occurs as retinol (the animal form) and beta-carotene (the vegetable form). In supplements, retinol comes from fish oil, while most beta-carotene supplements are synthetic.*

Evidence exists that women who eat more beta-carotene[16] or retinol[17] have a lower risk of breast cancer; although both are thought to potentially reduce cancer risk, most evidence suggests that beta-carotene is more protective. For example, a Canadian study found that the more beta-carotene women reported in their diets, the less their mammograms revealed findings suggestive of increased cancer risk.[18] When these same researchers looked for a similar pattern with retinol intake, they couldn't find it. A review of the scientific literature found four of nine studies reporting retinol to be protective, but ten of fourteen studies reporting beta-carotene to be associated with protection.[19]

The higher level of protection associated with beta-carotene appears to exist because it is a better antioxidant than retinol. (In terms of supplementation, this is fortuitous because retinol can be toxic, but beta-carotene is virtually nontoxic.) Women who eat

---

*Natural carotenes from sea plants and palm oil are appearing on the market. The palm oil carotene contains substantial amounts of alpha-carotene, a molecule very similar to beta. The little that is known about alpha-carotene suggests it also has anticancer activity, but we don't yet know whether alpha-carotene has a unique contribution to make.

more vegetables — the best dietary source of beta-carotene — have a lowered risk of breast cancer.[20] In fact, one study reports that Greek women eating the highest level of vegetables had a risk of breast cancer 90 percent lower than that of women with the lowest intake.[21] A Russian study also reported the same dramatic results, though most of the protection was found in postmenopausal women.[22]

Although these results are exciting, much of the protection derived from vegetables probably comes from constituents other than carotene. Compare the dramatic figures from the Greek study looking at vegetables with a report that combined twelve different breast cancer/nutrition studies and found that people eating higher levels of beta-carotene had only a 5 to 19 percent lower risk of cancer.[23] Even those numbers seem well worth the few cents a day it costs for supplements. The *Nutrition Reviews* article cited earlier shows that leading scientists in the field are convinced the association between carotene and cancer prevention is what researchers call "cause and effect," which means they believe carotene causes a reduction in cancer risk.

Like the Greek and Russian studies, a recent study done in Singapore found foods containing beta-carotene to be associated with dramatic protection.[24] This report found that the quintile (20 percent) of Singapore women eating the highest level of beta-carotene had a risk of premenopausal breast cancer 80 percent lower than that of the quintile eating the least carotene.

An interesting aspect of the Singapore study is the dramatic difference in risk between those at the top versus those at the bottom of carotene intake. The numbers look somewhat like the Greek and Russian studies mentioned earlier. It's quite possible that people at the very bottom of carotene intake are actually experiencing an outright deficiency. It's therefore possible these dramatic reductions in breast cancer risk are caused primarily by overcoming a deficiency disease. (In animal studies a beta-carotene/retinol deficiency will increase cancer risk.) If so, it suggests that many American women will benefit less from carotene supplementation than will women in poorer countries — American women are much less likely to have an outright deficiency.

The Nurses' Health Study supports this concept. Investigating exclusively American women, the Nurses' Health Study found that carotene (and retinol) supplements protect only those who eat inadequate amounts.[25] When dietary retinol and carotene were studied, only the women with the very lowest intakes had an increased breast cancer risk.

How Much Carotene Is Enough?

We don't know. I take 25,000 IU of beta-carotene to protect myself from a variety of cancers. (Beta-carotene is most protective against lung cancer, by the way.) Cathy takes 100,000 IU per day of beta-carotene. The research does not support the idea that special benefits result from high doses in trying to achieve primary prevention. Cathy's giant dose may be inappropriately high. The low cost, lack of toxicity, and the fact that secondary prevention might be different from primary prevention have affected her decision.

Beta-carotene is stored in the skin; if you take too much, you start to turn carrot-colored. It shows up first on the palms of the hands. It never affects the whites of the eyes. These simple rules will allow you to distinguish carotene coloring from other health conditions. At 100,000 IU per day for five years, Cathy's palms have begun to turn color. The change in skin pigmentation is not associated with health problems.

SELENIUM AND PREVENTION

For years, studies have suggested that the antioxidant mineral selenium protects animals from mammary cancer.[26] American breast cancer patients have been reported to have lower blood levels of selenium than do healthy women in some,[27] but not all,[28] studies. Areas of the United States with low levels of selenium in the soil (and therefore low levels in locally grown foods) have higher rates of breast cancer.[29]

Blood levels of selenium are higher in healthy Japanese women than in their American counterparts; as we've discussed in earlier chapters, breast cancer rates are much lower in Japan than in America. The Japanese get selenium from rice and fish, two staples of their traditional diet.

Compared with healthy Japanese women, Japanese women with benign breast conditions have lower selenium levels, and Japanese breast cancer patients have levels lower still. Those Japanese patients with recurrent breast cancer have the lowest levels of all. American women who are healthy, have benign breast disease, or have breast cancer follow the same descending pattern of selenium levels; however, all American levels are lower than the Japanese figures.[30] Authors of this research believe that Japanese women have a lowered risk of breast cancer in part because of their higher selenium levels.

These relationships between blood levels of selenium and breast cancer risk did not hold up when the Nurses' Health Study measured toenail selenium a few years ago.[31] In this case perhaps, despite the fact that toenails are generally considered a decent indicator of selenium status, the Nurses' Health Study researchers were literally looking in the wrong place for a link between selenium and breast cancer. Research has shown that toenail selenium does not indicate anything about breast cancer.[32] Researchers in the Netherlands, however, were able to show that women eating the lowest level of selenium appeared to have a higher risk of breast cancer than did women eating the highest level, and women with the lowest serum levels of selenium had twice the risk. Yet this same Dutch study revealed absolutely no link between toenail selenium and breast cancer risk.[33] (Due to the small size of the study, these numbers did not quite reach statistical significance).

Gerhard Schrauzer, professor of chemistry at University of California at San Diego and a leading selenium researcher, claims that dietary intakes of selenium are inadequate to ideally protect against cancer,[34] although people living in South Dakota, Wyoming, New Mexico, and Utah get so much selenium from produce grown in local soil that they might be an exception. Areas of the United States with the lowest levels of soil selenium are Florida, the Pacific Northwest, the Northeast, and the Great Lakes region.

How Much Selenium Is Enough?

Because we live in Oregon, Cathy and I take 200 micrograms of selenium per day, which probably puts us toward the top of dietary levels found in the studies cited above. People living in areas with more selenium in the soil might want to take less. Although no one knows the best level to take, reports of selenium toxicity from China suggest that problems begin at five times this dose.[35] The initial sign of toxicity is loss of thumbnails. This condition has not yet been reported from supplement use in America.

VITAMIN E AND PREVENTION

In a test tube, vitamin E prospects look great. Vitamin E has been reported to inhibit the reproduction of breast cancer cells and increase levels of TGF-β — a cancer-inhibiting substance.

In humans, however, very little has been done to assess what preventive role vitamin E has. A ten-year-old British study reported that women who eventually developed breast cancer had lower blood levels of the vitamin than did healthy women.[36] But the same researchers decided that reduced levels of vitamin E may be caused by the cancer, rather than vice versa.[37] The Singapore study mentioned in the beta-carotene discussion found that women who get more vitamin E from their diets have a reduced risk of breast cancer; but due to an inadequate number of patients, this difference wasn't statistically significant.[38] One Finnish trial found the combination of low serum levels of both vitamin E and selenium associated with a ten-fold increase in breast cancer risk, though lowered levels of vitamin E alone did not correlate.[39] And although Canadian researchers have found lower vitamin E levels in patients,[40] French and Italian scientists reported the exact opposite.[41] An American study reported dietary E protective, but less so when supplements were added in.[42] It should almost go without saying that the Nurses' Health Study did not find vitamin E protective,[43] but others have also not found any correlation.[44]

Evidence suggesting that vitamin E is protective against breast cancer is confusing and weak. This may simply result from the lack of available information, or vitamin E might not help — we're still not sure.

Because the vitamin appears to protect against other diseases though (particularly heart attacks[45,46]), both Cathy and I take 400 IU per day. Occasionally, an article discussing vitamin E will suggest that a long list of unlikely side effects might result from taking the vitamin. Most of these reactions have never been seen by legitimate vitamin E researchers. Most importantly, a careful review of the scientific literature has revealed that vitamin E is remarkably safe.[47]

A REVIEW OF POSSIBLE ANTIOXIDANT DOSES

Because no one knows what's ideal, actual recommendations don't make sense. I can only restate my personal choices. For primary cancer prevention, I take:

- 1,000 mg (1 g) vitamin C
- 25,000 IU beta-carotene
- 200 micrograms selenium

For secondary prevention of breast cancer, Cathy takes:

- 10,000 mg (10 g) vitamin C
- 100,000 IU beta-carotene
- 200 micrograms selenium

Before going on any long-term, high-dose vitamin or mineral regime, talk with a naturopathic or other nutrition-oriented doctor. Everybody is different and these differences suggest that each supplement protocol should ideally be custom-tailored to your body. Some of these differences you can figure out for yourself. For example, a 90-pound woman doesn't need the same dose as a 180-pound woman. But other differences may not be so obvious, so don't try to go it alone.

SUNSHINE, VITAMIN D, AND PREVENTION

A recent review of the literature shows that occupations associated with sun exposure and therefore an increase in skin cancer have low rates of other cancers. Overall cancer rates decrease as we get closer to the equator.[48] Researchers believe this evidence has something to do with the sun.

Parts of America receiving more sunlight have significantly lowered risks of breast cancer.[49] In the United States, it's surprising how much of the 80 percent variance in breast cancer incidence from low risk to high risk areas is potentially explainable simply on the basis of exposure to sunlight. The same pattern of more sun and less breast cancer has also been documented in the former Soviet Union.[50] Air pollutants, which limit the amount of sunlight that can be received, have been linked with breast cancer risks in Canada.[51]

As you may know, when sunlight hits our skin, vitamin D is made. After the vitamin D is synthesized, it travels to the liver and the kidneys for alterations that activate the vitamin (activated vitamin D). The final product is so powerful scientists consider it a hormone.

Receptors to activated vitamin D have been found in cancerous breast tumors. Initially, the presence of these receptors didn't appear to correlate with anything else.[52] In 1989, though, British researchers discovered that patients with higher levels of these receptors have a significantly better prognosis than do patients without them.[53] These scientists also gave activated vitamin D to rats; the result was an inhibition of mammary cancer growth.

When an activated form of vitamin D was applied topically to the skin of patients with advanced breast cancers, it led to a reduction in the size of tumors in women who had the special vitamin D receptors.[54] Lymphoma patients with vitamin D receptors have gone into remission when given activated vitamin D.[55]

What does this mean for you? First, it suggests that as long as you avoid burning, getting some fresh air might not be a bad idea. You might even take that Hawaiian vacation you always dreamt of (for medicinal purposes only, of course). We have become so concerned about increasing skin cancer risks that many of us simply avoid the sun or use sun-blockers routinely. The review mentioned earlier shows that sun-induced skin cancer deaths in the United States are far outnumbered by the apparent increase in other cancers (including breast) associated with decreased sun exposure. Nothing we've said here should be interpreted as an invitation to burn. Rather, allowing yourself some outdoor time without full sunscreen use appears sensible.

Does supplemental vitamin D make sense? One study has looked at dietary D levels and found no correlation with breast cancer;[56] but we would expect that dietary vitamin D would not correlate with breast cancer protection because vitamin D in the diet comes mainly from foods associated with higher breast cancer risk, including milk, butter, and cheese. The expense and effort that went into this senseless piece of research could have been avoided with a little common sense.

The supplemental activated vitamin D used in research articles and found to be potentially useful in cancer treatment is not available over the counter. The prescription form is much more powerful. Nothing is known about regular vitamin D and breast cancer. Despite this lack of knowledge, logic suggests that taking nonprescription vitamin D might have a preventive effect, because exposure to sunshine increases levels of the same form of vitamin D found in health food stores.

How Much Vitamin D Is Enough?

We don't know. If you live in San Diego or Miami, don't think about supplementing vitamin D. Go outdoors. But if you're in Portland with Cathy and me or other places as far north, it might not be such a bad idea to supplement, particularly in the winter. If you avoid dairy products, supplementing 400 IU for primary prevention or 800 IU for secondary prevention might be reasonable. Make sure that you don't supplement 800 IU in addition to a multivitamin that has another 400 IU or in addition to cod liver oil, which has much higher levels yet. In other words, 800 IU is meant as a total supplemental dose for people avoiding dairy products and living in areas of limited sunlight who already have a breast cancer diagnosis.

I find the evidence for supplemental D to be so preliminary that, frankly, I'm not taking any yet, though I avoid the use of sunscreen (which for me is no big deal because I don't burn easily). Cathy's D comes from her regular multivitamin.

Can Vitamin D Be Toxic?

Vitamin D can be extremely toxic at high levels, so "the more the merrier" attitude some people take with beta-carotene is definitely not appropriate here. Too much vitamin D can make people deaf or blind and can cause twenty other problems no one needs. On the other hand, increasing sun exposure does not cause the body to make too much D; when enough is synthesized, the body cleverly shuts off the process.

IRON AND CANCER

People who are iron-deficient need iron supplements. The first indicator of deficiency is usually fatigue. Keep in mind that the stress of a cancer diagnosis can also make you tired, as can chemotherapy, a lack of sleep, low thyroid function, infection, and a host of other problems. In other words, being tired is not synonymous with iron deficiency. If you feel as if you're dragging around, have your doctor investigate. Fortunately, the lab tests for monitoring iron status are excellent and, when used properly, leave little room for guesswork.

If you are not iron-deficient (many premenopausal women and the vast majority of postmenopausal women are not) *you should not take iron supplements — not even multivitamin/mineral supplements containing iron.*

In animals, iron increases tumor growth.[57] The same relationship exists when we look specifically at animal mammary cancers.[58] Iron-depleted women have a low risk of cancer.[59] Likewise, women (and men) with high levels of iron are reported to have increased cancer risks.[60] In fact, scientists are now studying whether removing iron from the body will become a cancer therapy of the future.[61]

The tie between iron and cancer makes sense because this mineral can act as a "pro-oxidant" — the opposite of the antioxidants discussed earlier. In other words, under certain circumstances, iron can create free radicals, which have been linked with breast cancer. Until more is known, don't supplement unless you're clearly iron-deficient. See Appendix D for a list of companies selling multivitamin/minerals without iron.

I avoid iron supplements completely, because I'm not deficient. Cathy is premenopausal and has a tendency to become iron-deficient. In fact, if she avoids all iron supplements she feels tired after a few months. She alternates, taking one iron-containing multivitamin/mineral pill for every two iron-free pills. By trial and error, she has found that taking any less iron leads to fatigue caused by iron-deficiency.

On the other hand, lab tests have shown us that reducing Cathy's iron intake to these low levels results in relatively poor iron status — which is actually what we're hoping for — poor, but not quite poor enough to feel tired. She doesn't totally avoid iron because the fatigue of iron deficiency interferes with quality of life. But remember, if you're not tired, you probably don't need any supplemental iron.

Ironically, you may increase your risk of becoming iron-deficient if you change your diet on the basis of the information provided in Chapter 12. The iron in red meat and poultry is better absorbed than is the iron from green vegetables or grain. Some nutrition-oriented doctors have speculated that the reason vegetarians have less cancer may partially be due to poor iron status. In any case, such a change in diet for some women will lead to iron deficiency to the point where supplementation is needed.

The bottom line here is simple: If you feel tired, see your doctor. If you don't, stay away from all iron supplements, even those hidden in multivitamin/mineral pills.

EXOTIC SUPPLEMENTS

Sometimes people try to sell cancer patients all kinds of extraordinary products. Anticancer substances found in garlic, broccoli, green tea, cauliflower, soybeans, and cabbage are beginning to appear on labels in the health food stores. D-glucaric acid, glucosinolates, indole-3-carbinol, sulforaphane, limonene, perillyl alcohol, Bowman-Birk inhibitor, and genistein are names that will be appearing on labels in the next few years (see Chapter 12). Some are beginning to show up already.

Less is known about these anticancer supplements than about those discussed so far, though they all show anticancer activity in test tubes and in animals. Doses currently found in pills typically don't exceed what can be obtained from real food. In fact, some of the doses found in the health food store are actually much lower than you'd get by eating vegetables. The pills cost more and don't taste as good. Therefore, until more is known, Cathy and I still get these substances from real food (see Chapter 12). At the moment, the substances appear to be at least safe and are beginning to look promising, albeit at higher doses than in the pills now on the shelf.

Sometimes, health food stores will sell "super-antioxidants" — products that include exotic names like "N-acetylcysteine," "epigallocatechin gallate," and "Coenzyme Q10." Virtually all of them except "S.O.D." ("superoxide dismutase") have legitimate antioxidant activity when taken orally by humans. In terms of cancer risks, however, we know virtually nothing about them. They are also more expensive than the common antioxidants. As yet, we have no reason to believe they would necessarily do more to reduce cancer risk than would the cheaper, more familiar supplements discussed earlier in the chapter.

References

1. Ernst, E. Complementary medicine. *Lancet* 1993;341:1626.

2. Just the facts. *Nutrition Action,* June, 1992, p. 2.

3. Malins, D. C., et al. The etiology of breast cancer: characteristic alternations in hydroxyl radical-induced DNA base lesions during oncogenesis with potential for evaluating incidence risk. *Cancer* 1993;71:3036–43.

4. Block, G. The data support a role for antioxidants in reducing cancer risk. *Nutr Rev* 1992;207–13. [This statement was co-signed by fifteen leading American scientists, including Bruce Ames, Elizabeth Barrett-Connor, and Richard Shekelle.]

5. Heenan, J. *Myths of vitamins.* HEW Publication No. (FDA) 1977;77–2047.

6. Centers for Disease Control. Analysis of L-tryptophan for etiology of eosinophilia-myalgia syndrome. *JAMA* 1990;264:1610.

7. Slutsker, L., et al. Eosinophilia-myalgia syndrome associated with exposure to tryptophan from a single manufacturer. *JAMA* 1990;264:213–7.

8. Collin, J. Tryptophan blamed, not contamination, for 19 deaths, 1500 illnesses—FDA coverup of information encourages hysteria. *Townsend Letter for Doctors* May, 1990; #82, pp. 245,252.

9. U.S. Department of Health and Human Services, Public Health Service, Centers for Disease Control, Atlanta. Recommendations for the use of folic acid to reduce the number of cases of spina bifida and other neural tube defects. *MMWR* 1992;41(RR–14):1–7.

10. Williams, L. FDA steps up effort to control vitamin claims. *New York Times,* National section, August 9, 1992, p. 1.

11. Howe, G. R., et al. Dietary factors and risk of breast cancer: combined analysis of 12 case-control studies. *J Natl Cancer Inst* 1990;82:561–9.

12. Taioli, E., et al. Dietary habits and breast cancer: a comparative study of United States and Italian data. *Nutr Cancer* 1991;16:259–65.

13. Hunter, D. J., et al. A prospective study of the intake of vitamins C, E, and the risk of breast cancer. *N Engl J Med* 1993;329:234–40.

14. Garland, M., et al. Antioxidant micronutrients and breast cancer. *J Am Coll Nutr* 1993;12:400–11 [review].

15. Block, G. Vitamin C and cancer prevention: the epidemiologic evidence. *Am J Clin Nutr* 1991:53:270S–82S.

16. Rohan, T. E., et al. A population-based case-control study of diet and breast cancer in Australia. *Am J Epidemiol* 1988;128:478–9.

17. Graham, S., et al. Diet in the epidemiology of breast cancer. *Am J Epidemiol* 1982;116:68–75.

18. Brisson, J., et al. Diet, mammographic features of breast tissue, and breast cancer risk. *Am J Epidemiol* 1989;130:14–24.

19. Garland, M., et al. Antioxidant micronutrients and breast cancer. *J Am Coll Nutr* 1993;12:400–11 [review].

20. La Vecchia, C., et al. Dietary factors and the risk of breast cancer. *Nutr Cancer* 1987;10:205–14.

21. Katsouyanni, K., et al. Diet and breast cancer: a case-control study in Greece. *Int J Cancer* 1986;38:815–20.

22. Zaridze, D., et al. Diet, alcohol consumption and reproductive factors in a case-control study of breast cancer in Moscow. *Int J Cancer* 1991; 48:493–501.

23. Howe, G. R., et al. Dietary factors and risk of breast cancer: combined analysis of 12 case-control studies. *J Natl Cancer Inst* 1990;82:561–9.

24. Lee, H. P., et al. Dietary effects on breast-cancer risk in Singapore. *Lancet* 1991;337:1197–200.

25. Hunter, D. J., et al. A prospective study of the intake of vitamins C, E, and the risk of breast cancer. *N Engl J Med* 1993;329:234–40.

26. Ip, C. Selenium inhibition of chemical carcinogenesis. *Fed Proc* 1985;44:2573–8.

27. McConnell, K. P., et al. The relationship of dietary selenium and breast cancer. *J Surg Oncol* 1980;15:67–70.

28. Willett, W. C., et al. Prediagnostic serum selenium and risk of cancer. *Lancet* 1983;ii:130–4.

29. Foster, H. D. Selenium and cancer prevention. *J Nutr* 1988;118:237 [letter].

30. Schrauzer, G. N., et al. Selenium in the blood of Japanese and American women with and without breast cancer and fibrocystic disease. *Jpn J Cancer Res (Gann)* 1985;76:374–7.

31. Hunter, D. J., et al. A prospective study of selenium status and breast cancer risk. *JAMA* 1990;264:1128–31.

32. Van Noord, P. A. H., et al. Selenium levels in nails of premenopausal breast cancer patients assessed prediagnostically in a cohort-nested case-referent study among women screened in the DOM project. *Int J Epidemiol* 1987;16:318–22.

33. van't Veer, P., et al. Selenium in diet, blood and toenails in relation to breast cancer: a case-control study. *Am J Epidemiol* 1990;131:987–94.

34. Liebman, B. Must we rely on supplements to get enough? *Nutrition Action* December, 1983, p. 5–10.

35. Yang, G., et al. Endemic selenium intoxication of humans in China. *Am J Clin Nutr* 1983;37:872–81.

36. Wald, N. J., et al. Plasma retinol, β-carotene and vitamin E levels in relation to the future risk of breast cancer. *Br J Cancer* 1984;49:321–4.

37. Wald, N. J. et al. Serum vitamin E and subsequent risk of cancer. *Br J Cancer* 1987;56:69–72.

38. Lee, H. P., et al. Dietary effects on breast-cancer risk in Singapore. *Lancet* 1991;337:1197–1200.

39. Knekt, P. Serum vitamin E level and risk of female cancers. *Int J Epidemiol* 1988;17:281–6.

40. Basu, T. K., et al. Serum vitamins A and E, β-carotene, and selenium in patients with breast cancer. *J Am Coll Nutr* 1989;8:524–8.

41. Gerber, M., et al. Liposoluble vitamins and lipid parameters in breast cancer. A joint study in northern Italy and southern France. *Int J Cancer* 1988; 42:489–94.

42. London, S. J., et al. Carotenoids, retinol, and vitamin E and risk of proliferative benign breast disease and breast cancer. *Cancer Causes and Control* 1992;3:503–12.

43. Hunter, D. J., et al. A prospective study of the intake of vitamins C, E, and the risk of breast cancer. *N Engl J Med* 1993;329:234–40.

44. Gerber, M., et al. Relationship between vitamin E and polyunsaturated fatty acids in breast cancer. *Cancer* 1989;64:2347–53.

45. Stampfer, M. J., et al. Vitamin E consumption and the risk of coronary disease in women. *N Engl J Med* 1993;328:1444–9.

46. Rimm, E. B., et al. Vitamin E consumption and the risk of coronary heart disease in men. *N Engl J Med* 1993;328:1450–6.

47. Bendich, A., and L. J. Cachlin. Safety of oral intake of vitamin E. *Am J Clin Nutr* 1988;48:612–9.

48. Ainsleigh, H. G. Beneficial effects of sun exposure on cancer mortality. *Prev Med* 1993;22:132–40.

49. Garland, F. C., et al. Geographic variation in breast cancer mortality in the United States: a hypothesis involving exposure to solar radiation. *Prev Med* 1990;19:614–22.

50. Gorham, E. D., et al. Sunlight and breast cancer incidence in the USSR. *Int J Epidemiol* 1990;19:820–24.

51. Gorham, E. D., et al. Acid haze air pollution and breast and colon cancer mortality in 20 Canadian cities. *Can J Public Health* 1989;80:96–100.

52. Freake, H. C., et al. Measurement of 1,25-dihydroxyvitamin D3 receptors in breast cancer and their relationship to biochemical and clinical indices. *Cancer Res* 1984;44:1677–81.

53. Colston, K. W., et al. Possible role for vitamin D in controlling breast cancer cell proliferation. *Lancet* 1989;i:188–91.

54. Bower, M., et al. Topical calcipotriol treatment in advanced breast cancer. *Lancet* 1991;337:701–2.

55. Cunningham, D., et al. Vitamin D as a modulator of tumour growth in low grade lymphoma. *Scottish Med J* 1985;30:193 [abstract].

56. Simard, A., et al. Vitamin D deficiency and cancer of the breast: an unprovocative ecological hypothesis. *Can J Public Health* 1991;82:300–3.

57. Hann, H-W., et al. Iron enhances tumor growth. *Cancer* 1991;68:2407–10.

58. Thompson, H. J., et al. Effect of dietary iron deficiency or excess on the induction of mammary carcinogenesis by 1-methyl-1 nitrosourea. *Carcinogenesis* 1991;12:111–14.

59. Selby, J. V., and G. D. Friedman. Epidemiologic evidence of an association between body iron stores and risk of cancer. *Int J Cancer* 1988;41:677–82.

60. Stevens, R. G., et al. Body iron stores and the risk of cancer. *N Engl J Med* 1988;319:1047–52.

61. Taetle, R., et al. Combination iron depletion therapy. *J Natl Cancer Inst* 1989;81:1229–35.

C H A P T E R
14

Lifestyle and Prevention

STEVE

After you've incorporated diet (Chapter 12) and supplements (Chapter 13) into your prevention program, it's time to look at lifestyle issues such as exercise, alcohol, birth control pills, and electric blankets. In some of these areas (like alcohol), definitive research clearly tells us what to avoid. In other cases (like coffee), understanding the relationship to diseases of the breast can get complicated. In other areas, like the effects of electric light bulbs, we know almost nothing.

In this chapter we sift through the research, keeping you posted on the good (sunshine), the bad (alcohol), and the ugly (attempts to downplay the risks of estrogen replacement therapy).

EXERCISE

Exercise appears to protect women from breast cancer.[1] Conversely, sedentary women have an increased risk.[2] Researchers believe that underlying these correlations is estrogen.

Thin adolescents have a delayed menarche — the first menstrual cycle.[3] Girls who exercise are thinner than those who don't; therefore, they have their first period later than do sedentary girls.[4] This means fewer total menstrual cycles — consequently, reduced exposure to estrogen.

Postponing menarche through exercise is natural. Before this century, girls frequently had their first period several years later than they do now. Menarche has been pushed forward by a lack of exercise and a high-fat diet. Using athletics to restore menarche to age 14 or 15 is simply a way to undo the unnatural effects of our current lifestyle.

Women who exercise intensely sometimes lose their menstrual cycle. While this may further reduce breast cancer risk, it causes bone loss and infertility, making too much exercise dangerous. No exact line separates enough from too much, but exercise-induced lack of menses usually affects marathon runners and underweight ballet dancers — not women who hike, swim, or jog a few miles a week.

Although most estrogen is made in the ovaries, fat cells also synthesize this potent hormone. Therefore, leaner women (with less body fat) have lower estrogen levels.

Encouraging your children or grandchildren to exercise makes good sense, but what does all this mean for you? We don't know whether women who become active later in life will decrease breast cancer risk. Obviously, it's too late to affect your first menstrual cycle. But reducing fat cells should lower estrogen levels, even if you are postmenopausal. Though the link between adult exercise and protection from breast cancer remains unproven, it's easy to recommend regular physical activity to improve mood,[5] keep off excess weight,[6] and reduce the risk of heart attack,[7] diabetes,[8] and colon cancer.[9] I expect future research will link adult physical activity to breast cancer prevention as well.

ALCOHOL

The link between breast cancer and alcohol has been explored using two kinds of research design. The first, "retrospective," investigates two groups of women. One group has breast cancer; the other doesn't. Both are asked about past drinking habits. Researchers analyze the answers to see if a significant difference exists.

Retrospective studies are often done because they require little time or money. But such studies depend on imperfect memories. Having a breast cancer diagnosis might influence how some women recall their past alcohol intake. Therefore, retrospective studies are considered weak.

The other type of research used to analyze the link between drinking and breast cancer is called "prospective." In prospective studies, thousands of healthy women are followed for years until a sizable number develop breast cancer. Prospective studies are expensive and time-consuming, but something is gained for the effort. At the outset, all participants report their current alcohol consumption without relying on memory. As a result, the prospective design lacks retrospective problems, and conclusions are more reliable.

In 1988, Harvard researchers pooled the results of sixteen previous studies.[10] This approach, called "meta-analysis," makes the results more powerful — better able to pick up the true relationship between alcohol and breast cancer. When the Harvard group focused on retrospective studies, two drinks per day were associated with a 40 percent increased risk of breast cancer. But in the prospective (more reliable) studies, the same two drinks were associated with a whopping 70 percent increase in risk. In most of the studies reviewed in the Harvard analysis, factors that might skew the results (like dietary differences between drinkers and nondrinkers) were considered, but alcohol and breast cancer remained tightly linked.

The Harvard group found that the relationship between alcohol and breast cancer was "dose-dependent." This means the more women drank, the higher their risk. Women in the prospective studies consuming one-half drink per day had a 20 percent excess risk, while those having three drinks a day had 100 percent higher risk than did teetotalers. "Compelling" is the way the Harvard researchers described the evidence supporting dose dependency.

Because of our high-fat diet and other factors, American women have a high risk of breast cancer — but being American doesn't cause breast cancer. Similarly, an association between two things like alcohol and breast cancer, doesn't necessarily mean that alcohol caused the breast cancer. Scientists are acutely aware of this. Nonetheless, the Harvard researchers believe their evidence is so strong that it "supports causality."

Since the Harvard analysis, some studies haven't found the link between alcohol and breast cancer[11–15] while others have.[16–21]

Meta-analyses like the Harvard report provide perhaps the best way to resolve these inconsistencies. In 1991, a group of six international research groups merged the results of their previously published studies in what we might call a "mini" meta-analysis. Like the Harvard study, this report found an approximately 70 percent increase in breast cancer risk when women had more than three drinks per day.[22]

Why Don't All Studies Find the Alcohol Link?

The Harvard study found only a 20 percent increase in risk if women averaged half a drink per day. A 20 percent difference is hard to detect between two groups with differing diets, genetic risks, birthing histories, etc.; it may easily be lost amidst other differences.

Even when studies are able to pick up a 20 percent difference, such a small variation will often be statistically insignificant unless the study includes many women. (A small difference between groups with just a few participants could easily be caused by chance.) Researchers tend to ignore results that aren't statistically significant, even if the only reason for the lack of statistical significance is that too few women were investigated.

There's another reason several studies don't find the alcohol-breast cancer link: People are notorious for inaccurately reporting their alcohol intake. Even a prospective study depends on honest answers. As those answers stray further from the truth, it becomes increasingly difficult to isolate a small difference in risk that might really be due to the level of alcohol that was consumed. Given these impediments, it's surprising so many studies have actually established the connection between alcohol and breast cancer.

Why Does Alcohol Cause Breast Cancer?

"Some alcoholic beverages contain carcinogens, and alcohol is also metabolized into . . . carcinogens in the body," according to the National Cancer Institute.[23] Alcohol also suppresses immunity.[24] Yet there is a more compelling reason for the link: Estrogen levels increase when women drink alcohol.[25,26]

Most breast cancer risk factors (including age at first menstrual cycle, age at menopause, dietary fat, etc.) also tie to estrogen levels. The alcohol-induced increase in estrogen is therefore most likely to be the primary problem.

When Does Drinking Cause Breast Cancer?

During early adulthood, drinking may affect breast cancer risk more than later on in life.[27] Therefore, if you're thinking of your adult daughter's risk, less drinking before the age of 30 may be particularly important. Nonetheless, some reports find that even drinking later in life is still associated with an increased risk.[28]

How Much Alcohol Is Too Much?

No one knows how much is too much. The Harvard study implicated half a drink per day. The international combined analysis, on the other hand, did not find a correlation at up to two drinks per day. It's likely that even very light drinking causes breast cancer in some women, but the relationship is weak enough to be missed in some studies.

How About Alcohol Substitutes?

Consider switching to alcohol-free wine. Nonalcoholic beer, however, should be avoided until we know more. Even when the alcohol has been removed, beer increases prolactin,[29] a hormone linked with breast cancer.

Why Hasn't My Medical Doctor Told Me to Stop Drinking?

Even if you already have breast cancer, some medical doctors don't feel the proof is strong enough to suggest abstention. Some of them simply don't know much about the link because they don't read the nutritional literature.

There might be another reason your medical doctor hasn't suggested quitting. Light drinking reduces the risk of heart attack — still the leading cause of death in American women. Therefore, some medical doctors actually suggest light drinking for people without an alcohol problem.[30] But if you're following the dietary recommendations suggested in Chapters 12 and 13, you probably won't need alcohol to protect you from a heart attack. Fortunately, the same diet associated with a low risk of breast cancer also reduces cardiovascular disease. Cathy and I each have a cholesterol level of 125 on this diet. Only 4 percent of Americans have levels below 140.[31] Heart attacks with cholesterol levels this low are virtually unknown.

Having Difficulties Trying to Quit?

For most women, giving up alcohol is not as difficult as making the dietary changes discussed in Chapter 12. If you dread the thought, consider calling Alcoholics Anonymous and discussing the issue with them. You might have a problem. Talking with an A.A. volunteer is often the best way to evaluate it.

COFFEE

Coffee has been linked with benign breast pain and lumpiness — formerly called "fibrocystic disease." Some types of "fibrocystic disease" have, in turn, been linked with breast cancer. Both relationships have recently been questioned, as we shall see, and it's clear that even if coffee does cause lumpiness and pain, it probably has nothing to do with breast cancer. Let's sort out what we know.

Many premenopausal women believe caffeine consumption increases monthly breast tenderness. Studies find avoidance of caffeine very effective,[32,33,34] slightly helpful,[35,36] or totally useless in reducing symptoms.[37] Coffee drinkers have an increased risk of benign breast diseases in some studies.[38,39,40] In other reports they don't.[41,42,43] Studies linking coffee and breast pain or lumpiness have been roundly criticized,[44,45] but so have reports claiming no such link.[46,47] Confused? So is everyone else.

If you are premenopausal and have these symptoms, there is little harm in conducting your own six-month caffeine-free trial. Remember caffeine is a drug; many people experience headaches due to drug withdrawal for a week after quitting. Once you've quit, the most likely "side-effect" is a better night's sleep.

Cathy eliminated coffee and, like so many other women, she's convinced her "fibrocystic" symptoms have decreased. She's also calmer and sleeps better. Here's a list of caffeine-containing foods:

- Coffee (even decaf has a trace)
- Cocoa and chocolate
- Many colas; even citrus-flavored drinks (check labels; caffeine-free drinks include root beers, ginger ales, and others — even colas — that are marked "caffeine-free")
- Regular tea, a few herb teas, such as guarana
- Some over-the-counter drugs (for weight loss, headaches, colds)

Avoiding caffeine may reduce symptoms for some women. But the cyclical breast tenderness and lumpiness experienced by many (premenopausal) women are not in and of themselves linked with breast cancer. When pathologists look at breast cells removed from women suffering from these symptoms, they find a multiplicity of conditions. That's why the nonspecific term "fibrocystic disease" is becoming obsolete. Some of these conditions identified by pathologists increase breast cancer risk significantly while others may not. Simply having cyclical breast lumpiness and pain doesn't necessarily boost cancer risk. And even if caffeine elimination does reduce these symptoms, there's no evidence that it affects the underlying cellular changes that sometimes do increase breast cancer risk.

While there is uncertainty about the relationship between coffee and "fibrocystic disease" and the relationship between "fibrocystic disease" and breast cancer, science has been clear about one thing: Women who drink coffee do not have an increased risk of breast cancer.[48,49,50] So coffee appears innocent, but one caffeine-containing beverage might actually help protect against cancer.

GREEN TEA

Green (Japanese), oolong (southern Chinese), and black (regular) tea all come from the same plant but are prepared differently. Green tea, the least processed, contains antioxidants called polyphenols. As discussed in Chapter 13, antioxidants are associated with cancer prevention.

The main polyphenol in green tea has the insufferable name "epigallocatechin-3-gallate." If you want to pronounce it, the "ch" can be hard or soft ("k" or "tsh"). Doesn't that help? No? Then let's just call it EGCG as many scientists do when trying to hide the fact that they can't pronounce the word either. Some green tea investigations study all the polyphenols, while others look at just EGCG. Careful distinctions are probably unnecessary — EGCG is the most active and abundant of the green tea polyphenols.

EGCG is anticarcinogenic in animals.[51,52] It even inhibits animal skin cancers when applied directly to the skin.[53] EGCG has also been found to stop the formation of carcinogens in humans.[54] Japanese who drink relatively more green tea have a lowered risk of stomach cancer.[55] Feeding EGCG to animals also lowers their cholesterol,[56] and human green tea drinkers have lowered serum cholesterol levels.[57]

Of course, much of the green tea research is done in Japan. Because breast cancer isn't a big problem there, EGCG research in breast cancer patients doesn't yet exist. Two unpublished animal studies report decreased mammary tumor size and inhibition of mammary tumor formation.[58] These results are quite preliminary. Nonetheless, I'm impressed that green tea and EGCG have been linked with protection from several cancers, and they appear harmless. For now, we can say green tea is safe and may prove protective.

Becoming a Green Tea Maven

Green tea can be found in supermarkets. Health food stores raise the price and call it "bancha." Actually, bancha is the lowest grade of green tea. If your town has a Japanese grocery store, you'll find many brands of affordable bancha but also other "cha"s with

especially delicate flavors and higher prices. It's easy to identify
the green tea — it's green.

"Cha" is Japanese for tea. Simply asking for "cha" in a Japanese restaurant, however, is not too cool; because green tea is so
revered in Japan, the Japanese say "o-cha" (pronounced aw-cha),
which means "honorable tea." In Japanese restaurants, if you ask
for ocha, the waitress will bring you bancha. If you're lucky
enough to attend a Japanese tea ceremony, the quality of the
green tea will be much higher.

EGCG pills sometimes labeled "green tea polyphenols" are
becoming available in health food stores. A cup of green tea contains about 142 mg of EGCG and more than 250 mg of total
polyphenols per cup.[59] Typically, EGCG pills contain less than the
amount in a cup of the tea. Because EGCG pills are more expensive than bancha and don't taste as good, why not just brew up
some honorable green tea instead?

Boil water, put a few heaping teaspoonfuls of green tea into
a small sieve set into the opening of the tea pot, and pour the hot
water through the sieve into the pot. That's it. Using lemon,
cream, or sugar in green tea is like putting mustard and ketchup
in coffee.

WEIGHT

By now, you might expect overweight women to have a high
breast cancer risk, keeping in mind that:

- Overweight is often the result of a high-fat diet.
- Overweight is often accompanied by lack of exercise.
- Fat cells make estrogen.
- Overweight in childhood is linked to an earlier first menstrual
  cycle,[60] and early menarche is an accepted risk factor.[61]

Weight and Postmenopausal Breast Cancer

Overweight postmenopausal women do have an increased breast
cancer risk, according to most studies.[62] For example, an Israeli

team found heavier postmenopausal women had 2.5 times the risk of getting breast cancer than thin postmenopausal women had.[63] Among breast cancer patients, those who are obese are more likely to have positive nodes.[64] Simply gaining weight is linked to breast cancer risk.[65,66] Overweight patients have a higher chance of suffering a recurrence[67,68,69] and dying from breast cancer.[70,71]

But not every study finds that overweight postmenopausal women have a higher risk. In Chapter 13, I mentioned that the Nurses' Health Study group couldn't find the link between vitamin C, vitamin E, or selenium and breast cancer prevention. They also couldn't tie dietary fat to increased breast cancer risk (Chapter 12). As you might expect, when the researchers looked for a correlation between obesity and postmenopausal breast cancer, they couldn't find that either.[72] Why their results are generally out of line with the work of most other researchers remains a mystery. Possibly, the subjects in the Nurses' Health Study, a group of American nurses, are somehow not representative of other women.*

When most of the research draws one conclusion, and a few researchers deduce the opposite, I look at the quality of the research. If that doesn't help solve the mystery, I do something naturopathic doctors are trained to do but conventional medical doctors are discouraged from doing. We give ourselves permission to use common sense. In this case, I observe the list of relationships between weight, estrogen, diet, exercise, and menarche listed on page 240. Then I note that most, though admittedly not all, of the research leans in the expected direction — overweight increases risk. I recall that women in Thailand, Korea, and other places with very low postmenopausal rates of breast cancer are rarely obese, and women from high risk countries are commonly

---

*For example, the Nurses' Health Study menopausal women were mostly in their fifties. The women in most other studies are older. Another difference might be that the nurses may know more about breast cancer risk factors than do other women; this could affect how they answer questions.

overweight. I remember that overweight has been definitively linked with high blood pressure, gallstones, heart attack, and other diseases. Then, using common sense, I decided it's appropriate to encourage early-stage postmenopausal breast cancer patients who are overweight to trim down.

"Of course," you might say. What's wrong with common sense? I can't answer that question, but it is clear that conventional medicine disdains it. Consider the following:

Since the turn of the century, naturopathic doctors have been telling their patients not to smoke. We noticed that few nonsmokers get lung cancer and that most lung cancer patients are smokers. Using common sense, we also understood long ago that smoke is drawn into the lungs, which weren't designed to deal with it. On the other hand, conventional medicine didn't discourage smoking until many years later, when the link between tobacco and cancer had been proven definitively. Similarly, it took many years to prove that infant formula was inferior to mother's milk. Until the proof was conclusive, medical doctors told women it was fine to feed their babies formula; after all, it hadn't yet been proven inferior. But anyone with half a brain could have realized that what was designed in a test tube in several years would not equal what nature had taken millions of years to custom blend. To this day, protective factors are still being discovered in human milk.

With medical doctors, the problem obviously isn't lack of brain power — it's the unspoken prohibition against common sense. Naturopathic doctors have never told mothers to use formula, because it just doesn't make any sense. Researchers now tell us that lactation also reduces the risk of premenopausal breast cancer.[73] Recently, we've been joined by conventional obstetricians and pediatricians in our support for lactation. These conventional doctors could have accepted our position long ago had they considered common sense a useful tool rather than a shameful taboo. In the long run, common sense and scientific proof (when finally forthcoming) usually sing in concert. That in itself makes common sense.

Is any form of overweight dangerous? David Schapira and coworkers from the University of South Florida College of

Medicine in Tampa reported that overweight per se didn't link to breast cancer; rather it was abdominal obesity (colloquially called "beer belly").[74] Initially, it appeared that these researchers might have uncovered a link similar to the one previously discovered with diabetes and heart disease — it's only abdominal weight gain that causes these health problems. Others have also reported that abdominal obesity correlates with breast cancer risk — but only with qualifiers like "in women with a family history of breast cancer,"[75] or "in heavier older women".[76] Other research groups have found the location of fat doesn't make much difference.[77] It remains unclear whether it's any excess weight that increases postmenopausal breast cancer risk or whether only abdominal weight gain causes the problem.

Weight and Premenopausal Breast Cancer

Overweight premenopausal women do *not* have an increased risk. Even researchers who find the link in postmenopausal women don't find it in premenopausal women.[78,79,80] Several studies have actually suggested that younger women who are thin have a "higher risk."[81] However, most researchers don't believe these thin women really have more breast cancer — just a higher chance of being diagnosed,[82,83] because it's easier to palpate a lump in a thinner breast. Studies investigating the link between weight and premenopausal breast cancer find that thin premenopausal women have smaller tumors, confirming the suspicion that they are probably diagnosed earlier.

The fact that overweight doesn't increase risk in premenopausal women remains a mystery. Other enigmas separate pre- and postmenopausal patients. American women have a greater risk of breast cancer compared with the Japanese, but almost all the excess risk is postmenopausal. There isn't much difference in the chance of getting breast cancer at age 40 between Japanese and American women, but the difference at 80 is enormous.[84] Researchers who have seen similar disparities between risk factors for pre- versus postmenopausal breast cancer have come to wonder if these aren't two different diseases.[85]

You might conclude from this discussion that it's harmless for premenopausal women to be overweight. I don't. Overweight still causes many other conditions. But even if your concern is limited to breast cancer, consider that every premenopausal woman who lives long enough becomes postmenopausal. It's common sense.

Fortunately for those of you willing to follow the dietary guidelines in Chapter 12, you'll probably find your weight decreasing without the usual effort. Cathy once weighed 155. Now she weighs 120 and seems to eat all day (but don't tell her I said so). When fat is dramatically reduced, the volume of food can increase at the same time that calories plummet.

SUNSHINE

Sunshine exposure increases the risk of skin cancer and melanoma, but it appears to reduce breast cancer risks. The link between sunshine and breast cancer prevention is probably a function of the skin synthesizing vitamin D when exposed to sunlight. Getting out in the sun is a lifestyle issue, but taking vitamin D is a supplement issue. I made the arbitrary choice to discuss vitamin D and sunshine in Chapter 13 rather than here. See pages 223–6.

ESTROGEN REPLACEMENT THERAPY AND THE BIRTH CONTROL PILL

Estrogen replacement therapy (ERT) is given to postmenopausal women to reduce both the hot flashes of menopause and bone loss caused by osteoporosis. ERT has the added benefit of decreasing heart attack risks.

In the past, women were given an estrogen-containing drug called Premarin. (The name derived from the source of the hormone: *pre*gnant *mar*es' ur*ine*.) But Premarin caused a sharp increase in the risk of uterine cancer. To reduce this risk, most medical doctors have switched to mixed hormones that include progesterone-like substances called progestins. Adding progestins eradicates the increased risk of uterine cancer caused by Premarin. For women who have had a hysterectomy, Premarin is frequently still used — you can't have cancer of the uterus if you don't have a uterus.

For the average woman, the benefits from taking these hormones (especially the reduced risk of heart attack) theoretically overshadow the increased risk of breast cancer[86] — at least most medical doctors believe so. But if you were at average risk of breast cancer, you probably would be reading something else right now.

What Does ERT Do to Breast Cancer Risk?

Consistently, researchers link most breast cancer risk factors to a woman's own production of estrogen. It should follow, therefore, that estrogen replacement therapy increases breast cancer risk. But individual studies have reported everything imaginable about ERT and breast cancer. Fortunately, we can look at meta-analyses from which a consistent picture emerges:

- Disregarding everything that's relevant (dose of ERT, duration of treatment, other risk factors, and whether or not the patient is still on the drug), a relationship between ERT and breast cancer cannot be found.[87,88]
- Women with an average breast cancer risk who take ERT for a short time (2 years) do not have an increased breast cancer risk.[89]
- Women who take ERT for a long time (8–15 years) are at higher risk.[90,91]
- Women who are at high risk* of breast cancer are at especially high risk if they take ERT.[92,93]

- Women are at higher risk of breast cancer while they are still taking ERT.[94,95] (The excess risk appears to decrease soon after ERT is discontinued.)

---

*For example, women with a history of other breast diseases or with a family history of breast cancer.

- Higher doses of estrogen (1.25 mg per day) cause a higher risk than do lower doses (0.625 mg per day).[96]

Does Adding a Progestin Help?

When a progestin is added to estrogen, the increased risk of uterine cancer caused by estrogen disappears, but breast cancer risk does not. A Swedish study found the addition of progestins did nothing to reduce excess breast cancer risk — in fact, there was an increase in risk associated with the added hormone.[97] A review of the research shows there is little reason to consider progestins safe.[98]

Isn't the Decision Clear?

If you've already had breast cancer or are at high risk of getting it, you've probably read enough to realize that ERT with or without other hormones is probably not for you. Amazingly, some doctors still haven't received the message. John Eden, from the Royal Hospital for Women in Paddington, Australia, and William Creasman, from the Department of Obstetrics and Gynecology of the Medical University of South Carolina in Charleston have actually suggested that many breast cancer patients need not avoid ERT.[99,100] A group from the Royal Marsden Hospital in England reports that ERT appears safe, but the breast cancer patients they studied were taking estrogen for only an average of 14.6 months — not nearly enough time to evaluate the results.[101]

Fortunately, most medical doctors won't prescribe ERT to women with a breast cancer history. The decision about taking ERT without a breast cancer diagnosis but with a family history of breast cancer or other risk factors is handled on an individual basis by most medical doctors. I think this is one time to "just say no" except, perhaps, in some women with osteoporosis fractures where concerns about osteoporosis may sometimes outweigh the risk of breast cancer — a decision that should be discussed with your medical doctor.

Can I Steer Around ERT?

ERT is an effective therapy, but the benefits can often be obtained elsewhere. My suggested diet in Chapter 12 should significantly reduce the risk of heart attack, as similar very-low-fat diets have been shown to do.[102] Osteoporosis can often be prevented and treated through other means.[103] Vitamin E is sometimes helpful in the treatment of hot flashes, though there has been no research in this area for many years.

Estriol, a little used form of estrogen, may protect against symptoms of menopause without increasing breast cancer risk. In fact, a recent review of the estriol story suggests that it might actually help protect against breast cancer.[104]

How About the Birth Control Pill?

Oral contraceptive pills contain estrogen and progestins, though the dose of estrogen is much smaller than is the level used for ERT. As with ERT, a look at individual studies reveals anything and everything. And again, the real answer comes from meta-analyses, which show that women who are on the pill for at least four to ten years beginning early in life have a 40–70 percent greater risk of premenopausal breast cancer than do women who were never on the pill.[105,106,107] Swedish researchers have found that women who took the pill before age 20 and were later diagnosed with breast cancer have tumors with worse prognoses than do breast cancer patients who started taking the pill at a later age or had not previously taken it.[108]

Cathy had been on the pill for many years, beginning as a teenager. It had been prescribed to control irregular menstrual bleeding. Obviously, if she had it to do all over again, she would not have taken it. She was a child; she was not given a choice, and the medical doctor did not warn her of an increased risk of breast cancer.

Most breast cancers in America are not premenopausal. Except for the risk of premenopausal cancer in women who were on the pill for years beginning at an early age, the oral contraceptive does not increase breast cancer risk. Therefore, if you had been taking the pill and are now postmenopausal, it can no longer come back to haunt you.

ELECTROMAGNETIC WAVES

Electromagnetic waves come from many sources, including radio and TV signals, microwave ovens, electric blankets, and virtually all other electrical appliances. Though they used to be considered harmless, they do penetrate the body.

Most researchers find a link between electromagnetic waves and leukemia.[109] Scientists in this field have only begun to look at breast cancer. But preliminary links between electromagnetic waves and breast cancer have initiated a raging debate exemplified by a recent exchange of charges and countercharges in the letters section of a respected biological journal.[110,111] Scientists rarely use words like "deceptive" and "cynical" or call another researcher's work "a wild goose chase." For the scientific community, "them's 'fightin' words."

A rat study has linked electricity to mammary cancer.[112] Several reports find that men who work around electricity have an increased risk of breast cancer.[113,114,115] The relationship may hinge on the effect of electricity on the hormone melatonin.

Electricity and nighttime light from light bulbs reduce levels of melatonin. But melatonin lowers estrogen levels. Therefore, a reduction in melatonin from exposure to electricity or even light at night might elevate breast cancer risk. Animal studies and some human trials seem to support the melatonin hypothesis, suggesting that exposure to electricity and even to artificial nighttime light might be risk factors.[116]

Of course, some of this discussion has little practical value. Even if electrical fields are proven to cause breast cancer, you can't stop radio stations from broadcasting, you probably won't "kill your television" despite the recent bumper sticker providing us with that sagacious advice, and Cathy is not about to finish her part of the book with a quill pen instead of her computer. On the other hand, Cathy and I do survive without a microwave; and were we to move, it would not be across the street from an electric power plant or a radio station.

A *Science News* review of the research found electric blankets may cause birth defects and miscarriages.[117] But a subsequent
attempt to link electric blanket use directly to breast cancer resulted in only fuzzy and contradictory information.[118] In this study,
use of an electric blanket was associated with decreased risk, increased risk, or no change at all, depending upon the circumstances. And none of these results were statistically significant.
They could easily have been due to chance — we just don't
know. But because the electric blanket has been tied to other
problems, Cathy and I don't use one. In fact, the ambiguous research was Cathy's justification for the purchase of a down com-
forter — a way to stay warm without electricity. We are, however,
talking major dollars for a mere blanket. Cathy's happy. I com-
plain about the expense, but confess that it's nice to sleep under
something warm that's literally light as a feather — well, many
feathers.

Because the relationship between electromagnetic fields and
breast cancer remains unproven, most medical doctors ignore it.
They make the mistake of assuming that anything not yet proven
must not exist. Until more information is available, we're playing
it cautiously. But we're not turning our lives inside out as a result
of these preliminary data. In other words, if you're as attached to
your microwave as I am to the computer with which I'm writing
this sentence, I'd wait a few more weeks before calling the Salva-
tion Army. Just try to keep a safe distance away when it's on.

ECOCANCERS

The word "EcoCancer" may have appeared for the first time in the
July 3, 1993, issue of *Science News* in an article by science reporter
Janet Raloff.[119] It may soon end up in the dictionary. EcoCancer
refers to cancers caused by environmental exposures that increase
estrogen activity. The environmental dangers include alcohol and
electricity, already discussed, as well as "xenoestrogens" — unnatural substances that have estrogenic activity, such as pesticides
(see Chapter 12). Plastic, a xenoestrogen source previously ignored by almost everyone, is reviewed in Raloff's report.

Certain plastics leach bisphenol-A, a xenoestrogen that makes human breast cancer cells grow in test tubes. For now, we simply don't know if plastic leaching is related to human breast cancer risk. As a precaution, Cathy tries to store food in stainless steel, unleaded glass, and cellophane — containers that, for practical purposes, don't leach anything. We often cook in stainless steel pans. We've found antique stores are a great source of funky 1930s glass kitchen containers. If you like green glass, you're in luck. It's readily available and still somewhat affordable. If you like blue, on the other hand, put some extra money in your checking account before leaving home. Better yet, learn to like green. Cellophane bags can be purchased from Seventh Generation, a company in Colchester, Vermont (800-456-1177). If you're environmentally concerned, virtually all antique kitchen glass gets recycled — it's worth too much to throw away — and cellophane is biodegradable.

Much of this chapter has discussed what Raloff would classify as EcoCancers. How much emphasis you place on avoiding potential environmental triggers depends on how you feel about the (mostly inadequate) level of available information. In some cases, as with alcohol, the link to breast cancer is so great, that I believe all women at high risk should act now. But who among you will swap her light bulbs for candles? Spike Lee tells us to "do the right thing" — usually good advice. But for most of these issues, the "right thing" remains unclear and, until more research is forthcoming, requires your subjective call.

References

1. Frisch, R. E., et al. Lower prevalence of breast cancer and cancers of the reproductive system among former college athletes compared to non-athletes. *Br J Cancer* 1985;52:885–91.

2. Vena, J. E., et al. Occupational exercise and risk of cancer. *Am J Clin Nutr* 1987;45:318–27.

3. Ingram, D., et al. Obesity and breast cancer. *Cancer* 1989;64:1049–53.

4. Frisch, R. E., et al. Delayed menarche and amenorrhea of college athletes in relation to age of onset of training. *JAMA* 1981;246:1559–63.

5. Martinsen, E. W. Benefits of exercise for the treatment of depression. *Sports Med* 1990;9:380–389 [review].

6. Hagan, R. D. Benefits of aerobic conditioning and diet for overweight adults. *Sports Med* 1988;5:144–55.

7. Duncan, J. J., N. F. Gordon, and C. B. Scott. Women walking for health and fitness—how much is enough? *JAMA* 1991;266:3295–9.

8. Manson, J. E., et al. Physical activity and incidence of non-insulin-dependent diabetes mellitus in women. *Lancet* 1991;338:774–8.

9. Slattery, M. L., et al. Physical activity, diet, and risk of colon cancer in Utah. *Am J Epidemiol* 1988;128:989–99.

10. Longnecker, M. P., et al. A meta-analysis of alcohol consumption in relation to risk of breast cancer. *JAMA* 1988;260:652–6.

11. Schatzkin, A., et al. Is alcohol consumption related to breast cancer? Results from the Framingham Heart Study. *J Natl Cancer Inst* 1989;81:31–5.

12. Schatzkin, A., et al. Alcohol consumption and breast cancer: a cross-national correlation study. *Int J Epidemiol* 1989;18:28–31.

13. Chu, S. Y., et al. Alcohol consumption and the risk of breast cancer. *Am J Epidemiol* 1989;130:867–77.

14. Rosenberg, L., et al. A case-control study of alcoholic beverage consumption and breast cancer. *Am J Epidemiol* 1990;131:6–14

15. Meara, J., et al. Alcohol, cigarette smoking and breast cancer. *Br J Cancer* 1989;60:70–73.

16. Young, T. B. A case-control study of breast cancer and alcohol consumption habits. *Cancer* 1989;64:552–8.

17. Richardson, S., et al. Alcohol consumption in a case-control study of breast cancer in southern France. *Int J Cancer* 1989;44:84–9.

18. van't Veer, P., et al. Alcohol dose, frequency and age at first exposure in relation to the risk of breast cancer. *Int J Epidemiol* 1989;18:511–7.

19. Kato, I., S. Tominaga, and C. Terao. Alcohol consumption and cancers of hormone-related organs in females. *Jpn J Clin Oncology* 1989; 19: 202–7.

20. Sneyd, M. J., et al. Alcohol consumption and risk of breast cancer. *Int J Cancer* 1991;48:812–5.

21. Ferraroni, M., et al. Alcohol and breast cancer risk: a case-control study from northern Italy. *Int J Epidemiol* 1991;20:859–64.

22. Howe, G., et al. The association between alcohol and breast cancer risk: evidence from the combined analysis of six dietary case-control studies. *Int J Cancer* 1991;47:707–10.

23. Larsen, N. S. News: study suggests mechanism for alcohol-breast cancer link. *J Natl Cancer Inst* 1993;85:700–1.

24. MacGregor, R. R. Alcohol and immune defense. *JAMA* 1986;256:1474–9.

25. Reichman, M. E., et al. Effects of alcohol consumption on plasma and urinary hormone concentrations in premenopausal women. *J Natl Cancer Inst* 1993;85:722–7.

26. Gavaler, J. S. Alcohol and nutrition in postmenopausal women. *J Am Coll Nutr* 1993;12:349–56 [review].

27. van't Veer, P., et al. Alcohol dose, frequency and age at first exposure in relation to the risk of breast cancer. *Int J Epidemiol* 1989;18:511–7.

28. Young, T. B. A case-control study of breast cancer and alcohol consumption habits. *Cancer* 1989;64:552–8.

29. Carlson, H. E., H. L. Wasser, and R. D. Reidelberger. Beer-induced prolactin secretion. *J Clin Endocrinol Metabol* 1985;60:673–7.

30. Kaplan, N. M. Bashing booze: the danger of losing the benefits of moderate alcohol consumption. *Am Heart J* 1991;121:1854–6.

31. Johnson, C. L., et al. Declining serum total cholesterol levels among U.S. adults: the national health and nutrition examination surveys. *JAMA* 1993;269:3002–8.

32. Minton, J. P., et al. Caffeine, cyclic nucleotides, and breast disease. *Surgery* 1979;86:105–9.

33. Brooks, P. G., et al. Measuring the effect of caffeine restriction on fibrocystic breast disease. *J Reprod Med* 1981;26:279–82.

34. Russell, L. C. Caffeine restriction as initial treatment for breast pain. *Nurse Practitioner* 1989;14:36–40.

35. Ernster, V. L., et al. Effects of caffeine-free diet on benign breast disease: a randomized trial. *Surgery* 1982;91:263–7.

36. Lawson, D. H., et al. Coffee and tea consumption and breast disease. *Surgery* 1981;90:801–3.

37. Allen, S. S., and D. G. Froberg. The effect of decreased caffeine consumption on benign proliferative breast disease: a randomized clinical trial. *Surgery* 1987;101:720–30.

38. LaVecchia, C., et al. Benign breast disease and consumption of beverages containing methylxanthines. *J Natl Cancer Inst* 1985;74:995–1000.

39. Boyle, C. A., et al. Caffeine consumption and fibrocystic breast disease: a case-control epidemiologic study. *J Natl Cancer Inst* 1984;72:1015–9.

40. Odenheimer, D. J., et al. Risk factors for benign breast disease: a case-control study of discordant twins. *Am J Epidemiol* 1984;565–71.

41. Lubin, F., et al. A case-control study of caffeine and methylxanthines in benign breast disease. *JAMA* 1985;253:2388–92.

42. Schairer, C., L. A. Brinton, and R. N. Hoover. Methylxanthines and benign breast disease. *Am J Epidemiol* 1986;124:603–11.

43. Marshall, J., S. Graham, and M. Swanson. Caffeine consumption and benign breast disease: a case-control comparison. *Am J Publ Health* 1982; 72:610–12.

44. Love, S. M., and K. Lindsey. *Dr. Susan Love's breast book*. Addison-Wesley Publishing, Reading, Mass., 1990, pp. 81–5.

45. Heyden, S. Coffee and fibrocystic breast disease. *Surgery* 1980;88:741–2 [editorial].

46. Jacobson, M. F., and B. F. Liebman. Caffeine and benign breast disease. Letter. *JAMA* 1986;255:1439.

47. Caffeine link to fibrocystic breast disease questioned. *Med World News* April 26, 1982, pp. 17–8.

48. Schairer, C., L. A. Brinton, and R. N. Hoover. Methylxanthines and breast cancer. *Int J Cancer* 1987;40:469–73.

49. Lubin, F., et al. Coffee and methylxanthines and breast cancer: a case-control study. *J Natl Cancer Inst* 1985;74:569–73.

50. Lê, M. G., et al. Alcoholic beverage consumption and breast cancer in a French case-control study. *Am J Epidemiol* 1984;120:350–7.

51. Mukhtar, H., et al. Tea components: antimutagenic and anticarcinogenic effects. *Prev Med* 1992;21:351–60.

52. Taniguchi, S., et al. Effect of (-)-epigallocatechin gallate, the main constituent of green tea, on lung metastasis with mouse B16 melanoma cell lines. *Cancer Letters* 1992;65:51–4.

53. Huang, M-T., et al. Inhibitory effect of topical application of a green tea polyphenol fraction on tumor initiation and promotion in mouse skin. *Carcinogenesis* 1992;13:947–54.

54. Stich, H. F. Teas and tea components as inhibitors of carcinogen formation in model systems and man. *Prev Med* 1992;21:377–84.

55. Kono, S., et al. A case-control study of gastric cancer and diet in northern Kyushu, Japan. *Jpn J Cancer Res* 1988;79:1067–74.

56. Hara, Y. The effects of tea polyphenols on cardiovascular diseases. *Prev Med* 1992;21:333 [abstract].

57. Kono, S., et al. Green tea consumption and serum lipid profiles: a cross-sectional study in northern Kyushu, Japan. *Prev Med* 1992;21:526–31.

58. Yang, C. S., and Z-Y Wang. Tea and cancer. *J Natl Cancer Inst* 1993; 85:1038–49 [review].

59. Yang, C. S., and Z-Y Wang. Tea and cancer. *J Natl Cancer Inst* 1993; 85:1038–49.

60. Maclure, M., et al. A prospective cohort study of nutrient intake and age at menarche. *Am J Clin Nutr* 1991;54:649–56.

61. Seidman, H., S. D. Stellman, and M. H. Msuhinski. A different perspective on breast cancer risk factors: some implications of the nonattributable risk. *CA* 1982;32:301–11.

62. Kritchevsky, D. Nutrition and breast cancer. *Cancer* 1990;66:1321–5 [review].

63. Lubin, F., et al. Overweight and changes in weight throughout adult life in breast cancer etiology. *Am J Epidemiol* 1985;122:579–88.

64. Verreault, R., et al. Body weight and prognostic indicators in breast cancer. Modifying effect of estrogen receptors. *Am J Epidemiol* 1989;129:260–8.

65. Ingram, D., et al. Obesity and breast disease. *Cancer* 1989;64:1049–53.

66. Ballard-Barbash, R., et al. Association of change in body mass with breast cancer. *Cancer Res* 1990;50:2152–5.

67. Herbert, J. R., et al. Weight, height, and body mass index in the prognosis of breast cancer: early results of a prospective study. *Int J Cancer* 1988; 42:315–8.

68. Tartter, P. I., et al. Cholesterol and obesity as prognostic factors in breast cancer. *Cancer* 1981;47:2222–7.

69. Fackelmann, K. A. Predicting the return of breast cancer. *Sci News* 1992; 141:239.

70. Boyd, N. F. Body weight and prognosis in breast cancer. *J Natl Cancer Inst* 1981;67:785–9.

71. Kyogoku, S., et al. Survival of breast-cancer patients and body size indicators. *Int J Cancer* 1990;46:824–31.

72. London, S. J., et al. Prospective study of relative weight, height, and risk of breast cancer. *JAMA* 1989;262:2853–8.

73. Newcomb, P. A., et al. Lactation and a reduced risk of premenopausal breast cancer. *N Engl J Med* 1994;330:81–7.

74. Schapira, D. V., et al. Abdominal obesity and breast cancer risk. *Ann Intern Med* 1990;112:182–6.

75. Sellers, T. A., et al. Effect of family history, body-fat distribution, and reproductive factors on the risk of postmenopausal breast cancer. *N Engl J Med* 1992;326:1323.

76. Folsom, A. R., et al. Increased incidence of carcinoma of the breast associated with abdominal adiposity in postmenopausal women. *Am J Epidemiol* 1990;131:794–803.

77. Sönnichesen, A. C., W. O. Richter, and P. Schwandt. Body fat distribution and risk for breast cancer. *Ann Intern Med* 1990;112:882 [letter].

78. Kampert, J. B., et al. Combined effect of childbearing, menstrual events, and body size on age-specific breast cancer risk. Am J Epidemiol 1988; 128:962–79.

79. Negri, E., et al. Risk factors for breast cancer: pooled results from three Italian case-control studies. *Am J Epidemiol* 1988;128:1207–15.

80. Hsieh, C-C., et al. Age at menarche, age at menopause, height and obesity as risk factors for breast cancer: associations and interactions in an international case-control study. *Internat J Cancer* 1990;46:796–800.

81. Taioli, E., and E. L. Wynder. Family history, body-fat distribution, and the risk of breast cancer. *N Engl J Med* 1992;327:956 [letter].

82. Willett, W. C., et al. Relative weight and risk of breast cancer among premenopausal women. *Am J Epidemiol* 1985;122:731–40.

83. Swanson, C. A., et al. Body size and breast cancer risk assessed in women participating in the breast cancer detection demonstration project. *Am J Epidemiol* 1989;130:1133–41.

84. Kelsey, J. L., and M. D. Gammon. The epidemiology of breast cancer. *CA* 1991;41:146–65 [review].

85. Stavraky, K., and S. Emmons. Breast cancer in premenopausal and postmenopausal women. *J Natl Cancer Inst* 1974;53:647–54.

86. Cummings, S. R. Evaluating the benefits and risks of postmenopausal hormone therapy. *Am J Med* 1991;91(suppl 5B):14S–18S.

87. Henrich, J. B. The postmenopausal estrogen/breast cancer controversy. *JAMA* 1992;268:1900–2.

88. Colditz, G. A., K. M. Egan, and M. J. Stampfer. Hormone replacement therapy and risk of breast cancer: results from epidemiologic studies. *Am J Obstet Gynecol* 1993;168:1473–80.

89. Grady, D., and S. M. Rubin. The postmenopausal estrogen/breast cancer controversy. *JAMA* 1993;269:990 [letter].

90. Steinberg, K. K., et al. A meta-analysis of the effect of estrogen replacement therapy on the risk of breast cancer. *JAMA* 1991;265:1985–90.

91. Grady, D., and V. Ernster. Invited commentary: does postmenopausal hormone therapy cause breast cancer? *Am J Epidemiol* 1991;134:1396–1400.

92. Dupont, W. D., and D. L. Page. Menopausal estrogen replacement therapy and breast cancer. *Arch Intern Med* 1991;151:67–72.

93. Steinberg, K. K., et al. A meta-analysis of the effect of estrogen replacement therapy on the risk of breast cancer. *JAMA* 1991;265:1985–90.

94. Sillero-Arenas, M., et al. Menopausal hormone replacement therapy and breast cancer: a meta-analysis. *Obstet Gynecol* 1992;79:286–94.

95. Colditz, G. A., K. M. Egan, and M. J. Stampfer. Hormone replacement therapy and risk of breast cancer: results from epidemiologic studies. *Am J Obstet Gynecol* 1993;168:1473–80.

96. Dupont, W. D., and D. L. Page. Menopausal estrogen replacement therapy and breast cancer. *Arch Intern Med* 1991;151:67–72.

97. Bergkvist, L., et al. The risk of breast cancer after estrogen and estrogen-progestin replacement. *N Engl J Med* 1989;321:293–7.

98. Grady, D., and V. Ernster. Invited commentary: does postmenopausal hormone therapy cause breast cancer? *Am J Epidemiol* 1991;134: 1396–1400.

99. Eden, J. A. Oestrogen and the breast. 2. The management of the menopausal woman with breast cancer. *Med J Austr* 1992;157:247–50.

100. Creasman, W. T. Estrogen replacement therapy: is previously treated cancer a contraindication? *Obstet Gynecol* 1991;77:308–12.

101. Powles, T. J., et al. Hormone replacement after breast cancer. *Lancet* 1993;342:60–1 [letter].

102. Ornish, D. *Dr. Dean Ornish's program for reversing heart disease.* Ballantine, New York, 1990.

103. Gaby, A. *Preventing and reversing osteoporosis.* Prima Publishing, Rocklin, California, 1993.

104. Gaby, A. *Preventing and reversing osteoporosis.* Prima Publishing, Rocklin, California, 1994, pp. 131–5.

105. Romieu, I., J. A. Berlin, and G. Colditz. Oral contraceptives and breast cancer. *Cancer* 1990;66:2253–63.

106. Thomas, D. B. Oral contraceptives and breast cancer: review of the epidemiologic literature. *Contraception* 1991;43:597–642.

107. Thomas, D. B. Oral contraceptives and breast cancer. *J Natl Cancer Inst* 1993;85:359–64.

108. Olsson, H., et al. Proliferation and DNA ploidy in malignant breast tumors in relation to early oral contraceptive use and early abortions. *Cancer* 1991;67:1285–90.

109. Coleman, M., and V. Beral. A review of epidemiological studies of the health effects of living near or working with electricity generation and transmission equipment. *Int J Epidemiol* 1988;17:1–13.

110. Jauchem, J. R. Electric power and breast cancer. *FASEB J* 1992;6:3016 [letter].

111. Stevens, R. G. Author's reply. *FASEB J* 1992;6:3016–7 [letter].

112. Beniashvili, D. S., V. G. Bilanishvili, and M. Z. Menabde. Low-frequency electromagnetic radiation enhances the induction of rat mammary tumors by nitrosomethyl urea. *Cancer Letters* 1991;61:75–9.

113. Demers, P. A., et al. Occupational exposure to electromagnetic fields and breast cancer in men. *Am J Epidemiol* 1991;134:340–7.

114. Tynes, T., and A. Andersen. Electromagnetic fields and male breast cancer. *Lancet* 1990;336:1596 [letter].

115. Matanoski, G., E. Elliott, and P. Breysee. Electromagnetic field exposure and male breast cancer. *Lancet* 1991;337:737[letter].

116. Stevens, R. G., et al. Electric power, pineal function, and the risk of breast cancer. *FASEB J* 1992;6:853–60.

117. Edwards, D. D. ELF: The current controversy. *Sci News* 1987;131:107–9.

118. Vena, J. E., et al. Use of electric blankets and risk of postmenopausal breast cancer. *Am J Epidemiol* 1991;134:180–5.

119. Raloff, J. EcoCancers—do environmental factors underlie a breast cancer epidemic? *Sci News* 1993;144:10–13.

C H A P T E R
15

Developing My Prevention Lifestyle

CATHY

Let's face it. It's no fun to give up pizza and beer. Even though I had come a long way toward developing a prevention-oriented lifestyle before my diagnosis, the modifications required afterward were still challenging. Steve covered many of the possible lifestyle changes in Chapters 12–14. You might have a hard time giving up alcohol, getting regular exercise, or taking lots of pills. But changing what I eat has been the most demanding lifestyle change for me.

Food has always been a major issue in my life, as you will see. Although it may not be as big a deal for you, most of us have difficulties making dietary changes. I believe it's possible to alter eating patterns if you truly want to and are able to get the proper support. This change may well require professional help from someone like a naturopathic doctor and/or a counselor. Get all the help you need. Perhaps reading my story can help you take a step in this direction.

EATING AND DEPRIVATION

If you're trying to prevent breast cancer or a recurrence, you may be considering *major* dietary changes, especially since minor modifications don't seem to help (see Chapter 12). One of the first things you'll probably confront is a sense of deprivation—

258

especially when you have to give up champagne on New Year's Eve, pecan pie at Christmas, stuffing at Thanksgiving, cake on your birthday, cake on everybody else's birthday, and junk food at all those times in between.

When it comes to food, I know a lot about feeling deprived. I struggled with food for years, starting to diet in high school and continuing well into my 30s. I gained and lost hundreds of pounds.

I am one of the many who has binged and dieted—the yo-yo syndrome. I was as impressive a dieter as I was a big-time binger. I succeeded on every program I tried: doctors' diets, book diets, magazine diets, Weight Watchers, Overeaters Anonymous, Weight Loss Clinic, and fasting. I had great self-discipline whenever I was on a diet. While a member of Overeaters Anonymous, I even kept the weight off for five years. But I always felt deprived. And, with every program I tried, I eventually returned to binging.

These approaches to dieting all focused on controlling someone who was viewed as out of control or defective in some way. They were all based on limiting food, especially the food I wanted to eat—what I called the "bad" foods.

Marriage to Steve was a match made in hell when it came to food. He was devoting his life to teaching people how to eat well while I was snorting Twinkies. My guilt was immense.

Surprisingly, most of the time I ate very well. I wanted to eat nutritiously; I saved junk food for the binges.

How did I heal? Counseling was my key. It gave me support and opportunity to look for the reasons behind my compulsive overeating and do something about it. I slowly started to have compassion for myself. This sense of compassion allowed me to decide to quit dieting even though I was at my heaviest. I allowed myself to eat anything I wanted and I didn't label any food "bad." To me, this meant I wasn't "bad" either. I later read Geneen Roth's *Feeding the Hungry Heart* and *Why Weight?* I discovered her ideas were supported by my experience.

The turning point came when I went to graduate school in 1982. I started each school day by taking the bus downtown, stopping at a cookie shop, and having a couple of cups of coffee with cream and two large double chocolate chip cookies. This was breakfast two days a week. On the other five days, I ate shredded wheat with raisins, a banana, and skim milk. Cookie Cabana was the treat that got me through difficult school days. Buzzed up. This is not exactly the diet Steve would have wished for me. But I wasn't binging. Over a two-year period, twenty pounds rolled off, and my body found the weight it wanted. Without dieting. Without any restrictions. During this period, I generally had one rich dessert five days a week. At home, I ate a very nutritious diet. No one was telling me how to eat. It was my choice.

So, I successfully healed myself (with professional support) from a serious eating disorder—in part by giving myself permission to eat anything. In the years that followed, I began to eat better. Changes took place slowly. I began to find that a ripe mango tasted better than a piece of cheesecake. I was still eating foods that didn't fit with my naturopathic doctor's recommendations at the time of my diagnosis.

Added to my fear about the breast cancer was the scare that changing my diet would lead me back to feeling deprived—something I had worked years to put behind me. I found this profoundly frightening.

I think it's important that a person doesn't feel deprived. For me, eliminating foods that increased cancer risk was a natural progression made easier because I had already taken the time and found the emotional space to resolve the deprivation/eating syndrome. If you are a compulsive eater, you will probably need counseling before you can consider an anticancer diet. If your current diet needs major work, you may not be able to switch in one fell swoop. Consider doing it in steps, and get professional help.

Today, I'm on a very restricted diet, yet I don't feel deprived. About a year after my diagnosis, several friends remarked on my great attitude toward my limited menu. It was true—I'd never enjoyed food more.

Looking back, I think this transformation happened in a series of baby steps rather than in one giant leap. The first step I remember taking involved alcohol.

One of my pleasures in life had been to have a drink after work—my cocktail hour. This was something I did to unwind at the end of the day, by myself, since Steve rarely drinks. When the weather was pleasant, I would have a beer and a couple of big pretzels on the patio. I might also read a book, pet my cat, or just look at the flowers. In the winter the same routine would take place in our Victorian parlor, often with a glass of wine.

I made a conscious choice to continue this ritual after the diagnosis even though alcohol was now off limits. I simply switched to bubbling mineral water or juice. It had been a special time for me, so why stop?

Letting go of butter was another big deal, since bread is one of my favorite foods—especially bread with butter. But I've discovered that really good bread (the expensive stuff) doesn't need butter; no more cut-rate bread for me. If I want to have toast, I put some spreadable fruit on it.

After the diagnosis, I slowly gave myself permission to have any food I wanted that fit within my new eating program. I actually added a number of foods to my diet that hadn't been there before. In the past, I never bought those outrageously expensive strawberries that come from the hothouses in January. Nor would I order extra sushi to supplement my already expensive Japanese dinner. The money would have stopped me. Now it doesn't.

In addition, new nonfat foods have appeared on the market since my diagnosis. I'm talking about nonfat cheeses, soups, cookies, crackers, tortilla chips, etc. I find many of these items at my health food store, but some show up at the supermarket or gourmet delicatessen. I enjoy being a food sleuth and discovering new treats.

I'm in the fortunate position of being able to spend more now in terms of potential long-term savings—expensive medical care for a recurrence I may prevent by being on such a healthy diet. I justify my more expensive food plan by thinking about all the other health problems I'm likely to avoid because of my wholesome diet—heart disease, diabetes, kidney stones, gallstones, hypertension, and osteoporosis, not to mention a variety of other cancers and obesity. Compared to the money I probably won't be spending to treat such illnesses, the price for the delectable foods I allow myself starts to seem minuscule indeed.

My approach may exceed your budget. Please don't get discouraged. There's nothing wrong with a simple steamed vegetable, baked potato, and broiled fish. If you want to add a little zip, consider being more imaginative than I've been. Vegetarian cooking without cheese can be delicious and inexpensive. Getting creative with beans, rice, pasta, tofu, and spices allows you to economize and still have tasty food. How about making your own bread from scratch? A friend who follows this diet and has a busy schedule often spends Sunday afternoons preparing large batches of food to freeze for several meals, thus freeing him from lengthy preparations during the week.

There's an old saying that the cup is either half full or half empty. I could be spending my days looking at the foods I've given up. I'd rather look at the half of the cup that is full of homemade bread, sushi, mangoes, medjool dates, salmon, vegetarian curry, blueberries, miso soup, Dungeness crab, persimmons, and fresh asparagus, to name a few of the foods that are healing to my body and spirit.

EATING OUT, EATING IN, AND IN BETWEEN

I don't like complicated rules about food. For me they trigger obsessiveness, defiance, and guilt. Keeping it simple makes it easier.

My general rule is to aim for two meals per day without any fat (except olive oil or fish if I want them). If I eat out, I allow one meal per day with up to a tablespoon of nonhydrogenated vegetable oil. This makes Chinese, Vietnamese, Thai, and several other cuisines possible. Some days I have three non-fat meals.

I eat mostly organically grown whole grains, fruits, and vegetables at home. While your medical doctor may scoff at this, remember the link between pesticides and breast cancer mentioned in Chapter 12. I eat very limited sugar, mostly a little honey.

Eating Out

One of the ways I avoid feeling deprived is to examine what I enjoy about eating and find ways to get it. I love restaurants. I like the ambiance, having the food prepared for me, and not having to clean up. Although Steve and I both cook, neither of us is a "natural." It's something we do, not something we love to do.

Hence, we eat out frequently. We choose our restaurants wisely and order carefully. Right after my diagnosis, I felt as if there were only two or three restaurants I could eat in. Now I can find something to eat in most restaurants, but some are certainly better than others. I stay out of fast food places. I don't frequent steak houses, but in a pinch I could manage a meal at the salad bar.

When I go into a restaurant, I am neither defiant nor meek. I'm assertive and friendly. I assume people will want to help me, and most of them do. When the waiter or waitress comes to take the order, I ask the questions I need to ask:

- Are there any dairy products in this? (Dairy in a restaurant is almost never fat-free.)
- What oil is used? (Frequently olive oil can be substituted.)
- What's the base in the soup? (Often a "vegetable" soup has a chicken or cream base.)
- What's in this sauce?
- Is this deep-fat fried or sautéed?
- Is there meat in this dish?

And then I make my requests:

- Will you please substitute olive oil in this dish?
- Would you please leave the cheese out?
- Can you make this without meat?
- Can you make this tofu dish without frying the tofu?
- Could this be poached or baked instead of fried?
- Please leave the croutons and egg off the salad.
- Hold the butter please.
- Could you bring olive oil and vinegar on the side for the salad?

If I think I'll be met with resistance, I preface my requests by explaining it's "doctor's orders." I have occasionally said I have cancer, but that is rare. Here in Portland, most restaurants are eager to help, but even in rural areas where there are more limited food options, I usually find people to be helpful.

Steve and I were at the beach one time in a small town where the pizza parlor was our only choice. We took a look at the menu and saw "seafood pizza." I asked the waitress if they could leave off the cheese. She smiled and said she didn't see why not. Granted, we did have to listen to them laughing at us in the kitchen, but the pizza was delicious. It opened up a new menu idea for us at home: We get a whole wheat pizza crust at the health food store and add fat-free tomato sauce, shrimp, anchovies, olives, mushrooms, Italian seasoning, and hot pizza peppers at the end. We've tried adding nonfat cheese, but prefer it without—like at the beach. Add a salad and you have a delicious, quick, and nutritious dinner.

I tip well, because I want the server to know I appreciate the extra care that has been given. Occasionally, someone makes a mistake and brings something I won't eat. I nicely but firmly ask that it be redone. I have yet to have someone not be gracious about it.

Steve and I like to stay in bed-and-breakfasts while traveling. I thought I would have to give this up because of the rich breakfasts typically served, but even here I've found most innkeepers very accommodating. When I call for reservations, I get specific with them about what I can eat for breakfast. I ask if they can possibly accommodate me. Only occasionally do I run into someone who won't. Then I go elsewhere.

My friends wondered how I would manage in Paris, sauce capital of the world. Very well, thank you. For two weeks I picnicked on bread and wonderful fruit for breakfast and lunch and ate one lovely restaurant meal a day. We don't speak French, so it was a challenge. A couple of times I had to scrape a sauce to the side and eat the fish underneath. But after Paris, I know I can manage anywhere; it's largely a matter of being creative and assertive.

On rare occasions, I have run into dead ends. Then I simply say, "I guess we can't eat here," get up, walk out, and go somewhere else. If being assertive is difficult or impossible for you, I suggest you consider taking an assertiveness training class or working on the issue in counseling. Such training will stand you in good stead for many other situations, not just ordering food in restaurants.

Eating at Other People's Homes

Educate your friends; martyrdom is not allowed here. Take care of yourself. True friends want to help. After my diagnosis, with each dinner invitation, I told our friends what I could and could not eat. Friends have become marvelously creative with standard recipes specially revised for me. One friend even makes a delicious apple pie with olive oil instead of butter or shortening and sweetens it with apple juice and raisins. Besides offering a tasty meal, such acts of kindness have helped me appreciate my friends' love.

Eating In with Friends

When we have friends over, I want it to be special. Some people define that as serving chocolate fudge cake for dessert, but there are other ways. I tend to go for an elegant setting—china, lace tablecloth, flowers, and candles. We have a lovely little dining room, so we do it up. When we bring out a fresh fruit platter plus medjool dates, Turkish apricots, or dried persimmons, everyone seems to relish it.

For friends who like wine, I suggest they bring their own and take what's left home with them. I don't mind having friends drink in front of me, but I don't want to buy wine. So I don't.

Eating in Between

What do you do on the run or when you're out in the country where there aren't any restaurants? Of course it's best to plan ahead, take a picnic, etc., but I'm not always that organized. My standard quick fix in such situations is to find the nearest supermarket, pick up some nonfat yogurt, fresh fruit, and bagels or the best bread available. It's not ideal, but it works in a pinch.

DEVELOPING A PREVENTION LIFESTYLE

Since my diagnosis, my primary goal has been to get as healthy as I can—physically, emotionally, and spiritually. This has led to the dietary changes I've just discussed.

Changing other parts of my life besides my diet has been an ongoing process. In Chapter 11, I shared some of the therapies I chose: psychological intervention, hydrotherapy, supplements, and herbal medicine. Integrating these therapies into my lifestyle required developing compassion for my predicament. Toughing it out with a stiff upper lip was not compassionate; I needed to make these changes more positive. In Chapter 11, I mentioned ways I found to take pills and tinctures that felt healing and ways to make the hydrotherapy sessions nurturing. I've needed to do this with prevention issues as well.

I had been getting regular exercise by walking, but now I include yoga as well, for both its effect on my physical well-being and its meditative qualities. I tried to start doing yoga when I was first diagnosed, but it was too much with all of my other treatment demands. Three years after the diagnosis, I began again, and the time was finally right. The work I did initially with relaxation tapes and guided imagery gave way to formal meditation four years later. I suspect things will keep changing. I see my work as staying in tune with what's working, letting go of what isn't, and being open to what might work better.

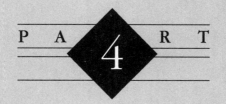

Living with Breast Cancer

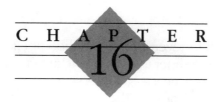

CHAPTER 16

Dealing with Change

CATHY

For most cancers, if you're disease-free five years after diagnosis, it's over; and often you can get on with your life as if it had never happened. With breast cancer it's more like Yogi Berra's line, "It ain't over 'til it's over." While many women live long lives and are never again troubled by the disease, the chance of a recurrence remains high for at least ten years and never completely goes away.

Living with breast cancer is a process that continues to challenge me in the most unexpected ways. I remain surprised and sometimes momentarily dismayed at the curve balls life keeps throwing me; recurrent fear has been one of those off-speed pitches. But fortunately, I also have a great deal of curiosity to see what will be served up next and how I can enhance my life with that new knowledge.

I thought I wanted the doctor to tell me which treatment option was a sure bet. What the two-year-old inside of me wanted was to be told exactly what to do so I could be a good little girl and get better. The doctor didn't have a sure bet to offer me. So, instead of being reassured, I was left with my fear and anxiety: Which treatment can I trust? Will it work? What's the right choice? Please, Mommy, tell me what to do. Please, Doctor, fix me.

Most of us have been raised to regard the doctor as the benevolent, all-knowing parent who will make everything right. Ours is not to reason why, but rather to follow orders and be rewarded with good health. Even those of us who have come to challenge this approach tend to revert to our childhood belief in the all-powerful doctor, at least temporarily, when we are faced with something as life-threatening as cancer — a regression based on fear.

When you're full of fear, the childlike part within you wants to find a doctor you can trust who will take away the fear. Perhaps you don't implicitly trust your doctor to "fix" you; you may have been reading or hearing things that discourage you from unquestioningly putting your life into the hands of your doctor. If so, you may doubt your doctor's suggested treatment recommendations, a dilemma that can produce even more anxiety. Addressing your fear may be a part of the solution.

In my case, there were many layers of fear. First, I didn't trust the conventional medical model because of past experience and because the scientific literature does not support many of the treatments offered. Much as we might wish it, for breast cancer there's no "tried and true."

Second, I didn't fully trust alternative medicine because of the lack of research. The thrust of my naturopathic doctor's treatment recommendations involved boosting my immune system in as many ways as possible so that it could more effectively prevent a recurrence. This made more sense to me than impairing my immune system with chemotherapy, but it still wasn't "tried and true." I wanted a sure bet.

The third layer of my fear was shared by the culture at large as well as by some friends and family members (even though they tried hard to hide it): The medical model is "real" medicine; alternative medicine is quackery. When my family and friends received word that I had opted for a holistic approach, including surgery but not chemo or radiation, and had chosen to do a wide assortment of alternative therapies, a lot of fear was stirred up. For example, my mother sent me a videotape that could have been a promotional ad for chemo and radiation. And a close friend took Steve aside and said he was concerned that I was being influenced by Steve to take an alternative approach rather than making up my own mind.

This last comment made me momentarily angry; nothing could have been further from the truth. A few days into the diagnosis, Steve had said he would supply me with research articles, go to doctor appointments with me, hold my hand, etc., but that he couldn't be my doctor. He said that if I chose some treatments under his recommendation and died, he would never forgive himself. He made it abundantly clear that if I chose conventional treatment he would support me 100 percent. Most of our friends don't know that I was interested in alternative approaches to health before Steve was. Long before I met him, I was eating brown rice, growing organic produce, buying meat (before I gave it up) that was free of hormones, and using vitamin E to heal skin wounds. Steve had been raised by a mom who put wheat germ in the brownies, and he was in revolt against "health" food when we first met.

I did not stay angry with this friend for long, because it was clear that he was only concerned for my health, as was my mother. Their treatment choices would probably be different from mine, and their concerns mirrored those of the culture at large. Fortunately, most of my friends supported my choices, and any reservations they had never reached my ears. I think this is important. To go against the cultural norm takes a great deal of courage. It's easy for other people's doubts to make you fearful of your choices even though they were made with careful consideration. When you're feeling two years old because of your fear, it's difficult to choose an alternative treatment or to reject any part of conventional treatment. After all, when we're two, we want "Mommy" to approve, whether "Mommy" is mother, friend, spouse, or doctor.

I thought I had finished with these first three layers of fear rather quickly and felt that I was home free. And then, twenty months after the diagnosis, I discovered that the third and most primitive layer of my fear — that only medical doctors could be "real" doctors — had come back in a more subtle way.

I had early on decided I wanted to be followed by a surgeon for regular checkups. Just in case . . . IT came back. Looking back, it's as if I were planning a party to celebrate the return of cancer. The surgeon was ready and waiting and so was I. All we needed was for the renowned guest to arrive.

The problem with being followed by surgeons is that they are trained to take one approach: to do surgery and to suggest chemo and radiation. This is what they know and what they are good at. When the patient doesn't get on the program, it's very hard for both the surgeon and the patient.

My doctor "supported" me in the sense that he was willing to do the limited surgery I asked for and was willing to follow me even though I did not do chemo and radiation. However, he was very concerned, and he expressed that concern at each visit. I was given a routine lecture that could have been entitled "Breast cancer is not like other cancers, and it can come back at any time." I knew that. I didn't need to be told every three months, and I didn't want confidence in my treatment to be undermined. But frequent check-ups and mammograms made sense to me, so I kept going. I suspect that if I got the lecture more often than other patients, it was because of his fear for me. He *believed* in the medical model, and I wasn't choosing it. When I talked about my alternative treatments, he tried to be supportive but couldn't quite pull it off. For example, I told him about the imaging group that I was going to at a local hospital (I figured that would be safer to talk about than my herbs — after all, it was at a hospital). He responded, "Some patients think that sort of thing is helpful." I wrote him a long letter telling him of my concerns and my need to feel more supported by him. I even bought him Bernie Siegel's *Love, Medicine, and Miracles,* hoping he could get behind it a bit and support me more, but he did not mention it at my next visit. I think he tried to respond and did the best he could, but it wasn't enough for me.

So I got another doctor. At least, I *thought* I got another doctor — a woman surgeon closer to my age. I remember being inordinately pleased that she seemed interested in finding out just what I was doing alternatively and that she wrote it all down. She also said a sentence or so in support of my meditation efforts. Give me a crumb, I'll make a cake out of it! I wrote my first surgeon a letter thanking him for his efforts and explaining that I was going to be followed by another doctor. The door was diplomatically closed.

Two and a half weeks after my first appointment with the second surgeon, I got a call. She told me that my mammogram was abnormal, no apparent cancer but a thickening of the tissue that was a concern. We would have to "follow it." And, oh, by the way, she just wasn't comfortable following me because from a medical point of view, she believed I "wasn't being treated." No, she couldn't recommend another surgeon. Frankly, she thought I'd have difficulty finding one who would be willing to treat me. She said if she had done the original surgery she would feel an obligation to follow me, but since that wasn't the case. . . . She would be willing, though, to see me until I found another doctor.

I was angry, crushed, hurt, and scared. (The good news was that I found out in a few weeks she had misread the mammogram. It turned out to be identical with the others and was no cause for concern.) And then my unconscious fear became conscious. It was hard to admit, because I considered myself way beyond it. I discovered that way deep down inside my unconscious, I still had the same attitude that the culture at large has — the medical model is sanctified, and alternative medicine is suspect. How could I not? This is the culture I've been raised in. I think there is no escaping this bias, even if you've been involved in alternative medicine for years, as I have.

I had to reexamine my motives for being followed by a medical doctor. The first motive was my fear that I wouldn't have a surgeon in case of a recurrence. Second, visits to the surgeon would be covered by my insurance; going to a naturopathic doctor would be at my own expense. But underneath it all was alternative medicine phobia. When I first went to my naturopathic doctor to have her look at my lump and she made a mistake, I was upset. When the radiologist made a mistake, I was upset. When the surgeon made *two* mistakes I was upset. Yet I dropped my naturopathic doctor and continued to be followed by the surgeon.

All of the knocks I had been receiving in my experiences with the two surgeons did help me look at my hidden prejudice and ask myself the question, "Why would I choose to be followed by a doctor who wouldn't be able to support my treatment choices, only my right to choose my treatment?"

My style is to act quickly once I become aware of something from my unconscious. However, in this case I chose to live with my discomfort for several months until I knew unequivocally what to do next. This was not easy. Being in limbo is not my cup of tea. I tried out a lot of different scenarios in my head and ultimately chose to go back to my original naturopathic doctor so that she could do routine breast exams and order mammograms for me. This doctor was a woman I liked and respected who had made a mistake that she admitted and then changed her practice protocol. This was a doctor who could actively support my treatment choices. I wouldn't have to watch what I said and could just be myself with her.

Now I feel that I have a treatment team: my naturopathic doctor in Seattle who prescribes my treatment, my naturopathic doctor in Portland who does exams and orders mammograms, and my medical doctor in Portland who is friendly toward alternative medicine and also does a yearly checkup. I no longer have to hide anything for fear of having my treatment choices undermined. I feel liberated.

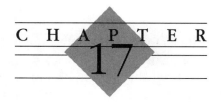

No More Headaches

CATHY

On the TV show *Thirtysomething,* the character Nancy had ovarian cancer. At one point, she said she didn't get headaches anymore — just brain metastasis. It turned out that Nancy was okay; but like her, I found that any ordinary ache or pain triggered thoughts of a recurrence, no joke.

For a year and a half after diagnosis, I was in perfect health. Everyone else got sick. Convinced that my treatment program was responsible for my great health, I believed I'd never get sick again. Then the flu struck, and it took me two months to fully recover. I began to fear the cancer would come back. If my body couldn't fight the flu, how could my immune system fight cancer?

A year later, I discovered a hard lump in my other breast and panicked. A mammogram showed nothing. I insisted on an ultrasound. Without any comment, the technician took the films to the radiologist. I was sure she had seen something, and it felt like forever before she returned. The verdict: a cyst. I began to breathe again.

One Christmas, I fell down the basement stairs and sprained my ankle. It healed in a month, but I had also reinjured my knees, and they did not heal. Years before, I hurt them while jogging and had to give up the jogging, as well as tennis and aerobics. But, with special exercises, I could walk, and it became a favorite activity. After my fall, I couldn't walk more than a block without shooting pains. Nine months later, I finally healed and was able to resume my walking — nine months of not knowing what was wrong. Intellectually, I thought I might have retriggered the old injuries. Emotionally, I leaned toward bone metastasis.

Two years ago, I felt three lumps on my scalp. The dermatologist assured me they were just cysts. However, I couldn't "follow them" through my hair and was afraid of melanoma. So I had them removed.

You might be saying, "She sounds like a hypochondriac." Maybe so. I've certainly become more aware of my body. Since the diagnosis, my doctors also notice more. After my optometrist heard about the diagnosis, she "discovered" a spot on my retina. She was practically sure it wasn't cancer, but just in case . . . she wanted me to see an ophthalmologist. The ophthalmologist had photographs taken of my retina. "Let's follow it" for six months. If it didn't change, we could assume the spot had probably been there since birth. So I waited another half year to be sure I wasn't at death's door.

My naturopathic doctor noticed two swollen lymph nodes in my groin. She wasn't concerned about cancer, but I was. I got a second opinion: nothing to worry about.

Before my diagnosis, I ignored minor aches and pains. Now I don't, even though I know some of my reactions are a result of fear and obsessiveness. In the process, I've developed compassion for myself by accepting obsessive preoccupation with health as a normal outcome of a cancer diagnosis. It's something we have to live with.

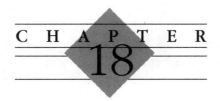

C H A P T E R
18

Getting On with Our Lives

CATHY

"Getting cancer was the best thing that ever happened to me." I heard that crap until it was coming out of my ears. Give me a break, I thought — I should be grateful for getting cancer? It was the *worst* thing that had ever happened. In time, however, I came to realize that I did have more of an opportunity to live fully with the diagnosis than I ever had without it.

After the car accident in Greece, I could have said the same thing. Driving off that cliff was a terrifying experience, but I was transformed. I recognized my mortality and was thrilled to be alive. I tasted every moment. The feeling stayed with me for months. Then, slowly, I began to forget.

You don't forget a cancer diagnosis. Awareness of a potential recurrence and death helps me remember the preciousness of life. The choices I've been making as a result have led to a richer life than I had previously imagined possible.

As a young woman, I had recurring suicidal thoughts; before cancer, I struggled with depression. The first few months after diagnosis were difficult, but since then my mood has been anything but depressed. That's not to say I've always been up, but I have been alive — and not by chance.

Shortly after my diagnosis, I attended a Bernie Siegel workshop. As an exercise, he asked us to imagine that today was the last day of our lives. The concept is simple, the implications profound. What do you want to do? What unfinished business do you still need to work on? For me, initially, it was my relationship with my sister, so I approached her, and she met me more than halfway. Our goal has been understanding rather than assigning blame. This has become an ongoing process. The result has been compassion — for each other and ourselves, and we are healing.

That was just the beginning. I began to use the "last day of your life" theme with all my relationships. I confronted problems directly and grew closer to some friends as a result. With other people, the problems just became more apparent. When a friendship was not working despite everyone's best efforts, the question became: If today is the last day of my life, is this how I want to spend it? I ended two friendships that were no longer nourishing. Although I have mourned the loss, I was also relieved. In one case, I didn't realize how weighted down I had felt until I let go. The relationships I've maintained have become more honest; the friends of a cancer patient go through their own trials by fire. As a result, friendships don't stay the same. People grow closer or farther apart.

Another side of "the last day of your life" philosophy is the living that unfinished business has kept you from. If I'm caught in regrets about dysfunctional relationships or about my past, I dissipate energy that I can use elsewhere.

My newfound energy and openness to redefining myself is reflected in writing this book. I thought, "Only creative people write books — not me." But Steve thought I could give the book life by sharing my decision-making process and the feelings that went with it. I was game. Writing has extended the limits of what I think I can do.

And, as it turns out, writing a book is the easy part. To get published, we had to face endless rejection. "I'm sorry. We just can't generate any enthusiasm for this project; there are too many popular books on breast cancer." Times twenty. Getting an agent and publisher takes perseverance and a thick skin.

Underlying my "I'm not smart or creative enough" assumption was an unconscious family legacy that also used to stop me: "Don't get too big for your britches." Somehow, success is equated with conceit. I'm beginning to dispel this belief rooted in generations of Puritan heritage.

Once again, as with diagnosis and treatment decisions, I have found that taking one step at a time makes it possible to move forward. For me, moving forward into the future has often meant working on the past. Your path will be different from mine. It should be. It's yours. Go for it.

We're rooting for you.

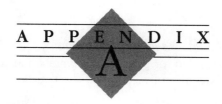

APPENDIX A

Making the Transition: Eating In, Eating Out

Getting creative with recipes and cookbooks you enjoy is quite possible. Start by avoiding meat, poultry, and fried dishes. Here are some substitute ideas:

olive oil	for	butter
nonfat yogurt	for	sour cream
nonfat cheese	for	cheese
dry-curd cottage cheese	for	cottage cheese
skim milk	for	other milk
olive oil	for	other vegetable oils
nonfat chicken soup	for	chicken soup

Here are some new cookbooks that will make cooking easier:

Vegetarian Cookbooks:

Jaffrey, M. *World-of-the-East Vegetarian Cooking.* Alfred A. Knopf, New York, 1992.

You will need to do some substituting here (olive oil for other oils and butter, nonfat yogurt for yogurt) and simply avoid some of the recipes (such as the deep-fried dishes), but there are many other delicious recipes to be enjoyed from India, Japan, China, and Southeast Asia.

Leneman, L. *The Tofu Cookbook.* Thorsons, London, 1992.

Substitute olive oil for the oil and margarine.

McDougall, J.A. *The McDougall Program*. Plume, New York, 1990.
This is a good plan for people who want some structure.
McDougall excludes olive oil and fish. You don't have to.

McDougall, J.A., and M. McDougall. *The New McDougall Cookbook*.
Dutton, New York, 1993.

Ornish, D. *Eat More, Weigh Less*. HarperCollins, New York, 1987.

Pickarski, R. *Friendly Foods*. TenSpeed Press, Berkeley, CA, 1991.

Pritikin, R. *The New Pritikin Program*. Pocket Books, New York, 1990.

Sass, L. *Recipes from an Ecological Kitchen*. William Morrow, New
York, 1992.

Macrobiotic Cookbooks:

Ohsawa, L. *Macrobiotic Cuisine*. Japan Publications, Tokyo, 1984.
Macrobiotic cooking has practically become a religion. Without
the philosophical overtones, you can still enjoy these low-fat
recipes.

Turner, K. *The Self-Healing Cookbook*. Earthtones Press, Vashon Island,
WA, 1987.

Japanese Cookbooks:

Downer, L. *At the Japanese Table*. Chronicle Books, San Francisco,
1993.
Avoid the deep-fried and chicken, pork, and meat dishes.

Omae, K., and Tachibana, Y. *The Book of Sushi*. Kodansha International, Tokyo, 1988.

Seafood Cookbook:

Grunes, B. *Skinny Seafood*. Surrey Books, Chicago, 1993.

Italian Cookbook:

Shulman, M. *Mediterranean Light*. Bantam Books, New York, 1989.
Use nonfat yogurt to replace low-fat and avoid meat dishes. You
can even make some of the desserts!

Italian cookbooks offer many delicious seafood, pasta, and vegetable dishes made with olive oil. Ignore the meat, dairy, and deep-fried dishes. Replace the chicken stock with nonfat chicken soup.

Thai Cookbooks:

Kwanruan, A., S. Aksomboon, and D. Hiranaga. *Thai Cooking from the Siam Cuisine Restaurant*. North Atlantic Books, Berkeley, 1989.

Focus on seafood, salads, soups, and noodles.

Neither of us has the time or inclination for elaborate cooking. So we keep it simple. Here are some of our basic meal ideas:

Breakfast:

1. Oatmeal and oat bran
2. Shredded wheat, whole-grain, nonfat cereals with nonfat milk or juice
3. Multigrain pancakes (available in health food stores) made without oil or eggs in a nonstick pan
4. Fresh fruit and nonfat yogurt, toast with spreadable fruit
5. Bagel with nonfat cream cheese plus fresh fruit

Lunch:

Sandwich ideas using whole-grain bread or bagels:

1. Sardines packed in sild sardine oil, olive oil (drained), mustard, tomato sauce, etc. with onion, lettuce, and tomato
2. Hummus (made with olive oil), sprouts, and tomato
3. Nonfat cheese and mustard or toasted nonfat cheese sandwiches in a nonstick pan
4. Tofu spreads — read labels or make your own
5. Tofu burgers without added fat

Other Lunch Ideas:

1. Fruit salad with nonfat yogurt
2. Nonfat soup
3. Noodles in fish or vegetarian broth
4. Dinner leftovers
5. Baked potatoes with nonfat yogurt

6. Baked yams
7. Salads, steamed vegetables
8. Rice

Dinner:

1. Soup and salad with nonfat dressing or olive oil and vinegar
2. Pasta (with fat-free tomato sauce or cheese-free pesto) and fresh vegetables or a salad
3. Whole-wheat, cheese-free, seafood pizza with fat-free tomato sauce and a salad
4. Vegetable stir-fry with brown rice
5. Broiled, poached, or sautéed seafood with fresh vegetables, salad, brown rice or potatoes

   ### Steve's special fish marinade:
   1/4 cup Japanese soy sauce
   2 T finely chopped fresh ginger root
   juice from half a lemon
   1 tsp oriental sesame oil
   6 cloves of finely chopped garlic
   cayenne pepper to taste

   Mix all ingredients. Pour over fish for four and let sit for an hour. Broil.

Snacks:

1. A little olive oil, cayenne pepper, nutritional yeast, and salt on air-popped popcorn
2. Fat-free crackers — by themselves or with nonfat cheese or nonfat cream cheese
3. Bagels
4. Fruit
5. Raw vegetables
6. Nonfat yogurt
7. Dried fruit
8. Fat-free cookies
9. Fat-free pretzels

Restaurants:

- Japanese: Avoid tempura, sukiyaki, shabu shabu, and other meat or chicken dishes. Most of the menu is fine.
- Thai, Vietnamese: Stick with the vegetable and seafood sections. Avoid deep-fried dishes. Some noodle dishes are meat-free.
- Italian: Hunt for meat-free pasta dishes and seafood. Confirm that the restaurant uses olive oil. Avoid cheese (which can easily be left off some Italian dishes).
- Middle Eastern: Avoid meat and deep-fried falafel. Confirm that the restaurant uses olive oil. Most dishes are possible.
- Chinese: Northern Chinese restaurant food is usually so oily that it's best avoided. Some meat-free nonfried Cantonese dishes (like vegetable chop suey) are okay. The abundance of fried (egg roll, fried shrimp, fried rice), meat (spare ribs, roast duck), and egg (egg foo yong) dishes make even the Cantonese restaurants a minefield of dishes to avoid.
- American: For salad bars, avoid the bacon, croutons, coleslaw, potato salad, etc., and go for the raw vegetables. Use olive oil and vinegar dressing. Many restaurants are accommodating to people with special diets. Broiled fish, baked potato without butter or sour cream, and vegetables without butter are often possible.
- Seafood: Swap olive oil and vinegar for the usual dressing put on shrimp and crab Louis. Broiled, baked, and poached dishes make good choices as long as the butter is left off.

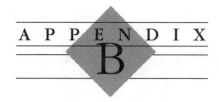

Guided Imagery/ Stress Release Tapes

Most cities will have audio tapes available in New Age bookstores, health food stores, and some regular music stores. Investigate! You can use them in a regular tape player if you have one. I prefer a pocket-sized player with earphones so that Steve can move freely around the house, listen to radio or TV, and not have to be quiet for me.

Some stores carrying such tapes provide headsets at the store so you can listen before you purchase. This is especially helpful because your reaction to the sound of another person's voice is simply a matter of individual taste. The tapes I've listed below are by people whose voices feel good to me. That doesn't mean you'll feel that way at all.

Lastly, I suggest getting tapes of varying lengths. You might want a 45-minute tape at the end of the work day to unwind, but a 10- or 20-minute pick-me-up in the middle of the day might be more realistic.

If you live in the country or a small town and can't find a store carrying such items, here are a few of my favorites and where you can write for a catalog:

1. Emmett Miller, M.D.

   "Letting Go of Stress"
   "Ten Minute Stress Manager"
   "Healing Journey"

   A catalog of tapes and an order form can be obtained from:

   SOURCE
   P.O. Box W
   Stanford, CA 94309
   800-52-TAPES

2. Mary Richards

   "High Mountain Meditation"
   "New Day's Promise"
   "Sunset on the Bay"

   A brochure can be obtained from:

   Master Your Mind
   881 Hawthorne Drive
   Walnut Creek, CA 94596
   510-945-0941

3. Robert Gass, Ph.D.

   "On Wings of Song"

   A catalog can be obtained from:

   Spring Hill Music
   P.O. Box 800
   Boulder, CO 80306

4. Kathleen McLaughlin, Ph.D.

   "Radiant Body, Radiant Heart"

   Information on obtaining this tape can be obtained from:

   Insight Seminars
   917 S.W. Oak St.
   Suite 420
   Portland, OR 97205
   503-223-9331

5. Bernie Siegel, M.D.

   "Meditation for Everyday Living"

   Tapes available through:

   Creative Audio
   Department BSS
   8751 Osborne
   Highland, IN 46322
   219-839-2770

   or

   ABC Audiovisual Enterprises, Inc.
   Department BSS
   500 West End Avenue #5B
   New York, NY 10024

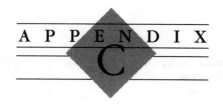

APPENDIX C

Food Sources of Antioxidants

Vitamin C
    broccoli
    peppers
    strawberries
    currants
    brussels sprouts
    cauliflower
    greens (like spinach, chard, and kale)
    parsley
    citrus fruits
    acerola tea

Vitamin E
    wheat germ oil
    nuts, peanuts
    seeds
    whole grains
    rice bran
    soybeans

Selenium
    seafood
    brewer's and nutritional yeast
    whole grains

Beta-carotene

- sweet potatoes
- carrots
- spinach
- squash
- kale
- turnips
- beet greens
- mango
- papaya
- cantaloupe
- dried apricots
- mustard greens
- collards
- spinach
- broccoli
- tomatoes
- nectarines
- prunes
- tangerines
- asparagus

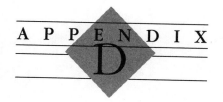

APPENDIX D

Iron-Free Multivitamin/ Mineral Sources

Nature's Life
Twin Labs
Country Life
Eclectic Institute*
Thorne Research *
Amni*
Tyler Encapsulations*
Pure Encapsulations*

Brands marked with an asterisk are available only through your doctor.

Questions to Ask Your Doctor
After a Cancer Diagnosis

Photocopy these two pages to bring with you to your next doctor's appointment following a cancer diagnosis. Write in your doctor's answers to the questions in the spaces provided. Refer to pages 27–28 to review what your answers may indicate.

About the Chem Screen (SMAC)

Are my liver and bone enzymes normal?

About the CBC (Complete Blood Count)

Is my CBC normal?

About the Chest X Ray

Is my chest X ray normal?

Pathology Report

How large was the cancer (as opposed to the size of the tissue that was removed)?

What kind of breast cancer is it?

What grade is the cancer?

Is my estrogen receptor status considered positive?

What is my specific estrogen receptor level?

Do I have diploidy?

Is my S-phase fraction relatively low?

Glossary

adjuvant chemotherapy: Chemotherapy used together with surgery or radiation to prevent the recurrence or spread of cancer. See *chemotherapy*.

adriamycin: Doxorubicin — a chemotherapy drug.

allopathic medicine: Conventional medicine. A medical philosophy based on the use of therapies antagonistic to diseases (as opposed to therapies that stimulate the body's ability to fight the disease).

amenorrhea: Lack of a menstrual cycle.

aneuploid: An abnormal number of chromosomes. See *ploidy status*.

antioxidants: Substances that protect the body from oxidative damage and free radicals. Examples: beta-carotene, vitamins E and C, and selenium.

aspiration cytology: Biopsy done with a needle rather than with surgery.

axilla: Armpit

axillary dissection: Surgical removal of axillary lymph nodes.

beta-carotene: The form of vitamin A found mostly in yellow and orange vegetables. Carotene is a more potent antioxidant than retinol — the animal form of vitamin A.

Biomedical Center: The Mexican clinic where the Hoxsey treatment is practiced.

biopsy: Removal of tissue, done as surgery (lumpectomy) or with a needle (aspiration).

Bowman-Birk protease inhibitor: A substance with potential anticancer activity found in soybeans.

BRCA1: A gene which indicates very high risk of breast cancer.

293

carcinogenic: Something that causes cancer.

carcinoma: Cancers derived from epithelial tissue (includes most cancers).

CBC: Complete blood count. Lab test done to rule out anemia.

chem screen: Common set of multiple blood tests ordered together.

chemical castration: Destruction of ovarian function by chemotherapy.

chemotherapy: Drug therapy; its purpose is to interfere with the replication of cancer cells, but it inevitably affects normal cells as well.

clean margins: When cancer cells do not extend to the outer edge of the tissue removed from the body.

CMF: Cyclophosphamide, methotrexate, and fluorouracil; drugs used in combination chemotherapy.

contralateral: The side opposite the breast that contains or contained cancer — thus with cancer of the left breast, contralateral refers to the right side.

Contreras, Ernesto, M.D.: A Mexican doctor who uses metabolic therapy. See *laetrile.*

cruciferous vegetables: Broccoli, cauliflower, brussels sprouts, and cabbage.

cyclophosphamide: Cytoxan — a chemotherapy drug.

cyst: A fluid-filled benign breast lump.

Cytoxan: See *cyclophosphamide.*

D-glucaric acid: See *glucaric acid.*

diagnostic ultrasound: A procedure used after mammography to distinguish between cysts and solid breast lumps; it does not involve radiation exposure, but uses sound waves to create images.

differentiated: Defined. Well-differentiated cancer cells resemble normal cells more than poorly differentiated cancer cells do.

diploid: The normal number of chromosomes. See *ploidy status.*

disease-free survival: Remaining alive with no return of the cancer.

distal metastasis: Cancer that has spread to another organ (other than lymph nodes).

ductal: Arising from ducts within the breast.

early-stage breast cancer: Stages I and II.

EcoCancer: A new term referring to cancers caused by environmental exposure to substances that increase estrogen activity.

EGCG: Epigallocatechin-3-gallate — an antioxidant associated with cancer protection and naturally found in green tea.

epidemiology: In terms of breast cancer, the science that looks for links between disease and lifestyle, nutrition, etc., by comparing one society or group with another.

ER: See *estrogen receptor*.

ERT: Estrogen replacement therapy — used to treat osteoporosis and symptoms of menopause.

estrogen: A group of female hormones produced mainly in the ovaries and secondarily in adrenal glands and fat cells.

estrogen receptor: Point of attachment for estrogen found on some breast cells. A positive estrogen receptor (or ER) status means that the cells contain a significant number of these receptors.

false negative: A test result which falsely reports that no problem exists.

fibroadenoma: A benign breast lump common in younger women.

fibrocystic disease: A term now falling into disuse; it has included a variety of benign breast conditions that appear as painful lumps which change during the course of menstrual cycles in premenopausal women.

fluorouracil: A chemotherapy drug also called 5-FU.

folic acid: One of the B vitamins.

follow-up: The length of time patients are observed in a research study.

free radicals: Substances that contain unpaired electrons and can damage genetic material, thus increasing cancer risks.

genistein: A substance found in soybeans that may interfere with a tumor's blood supply.

Gerson therapy: An alternative cancer treatment incorporating coffee enemas, and dietary changes.

glucaric acid: A substance found in some vegetables, including broccoli, that may increase the excretion of carcinogens.

grade: The extent to which cancer cells differ from normal tissue. Lower grades are closer to normal tissue than are high grades.

Halsted radical mastectomy: Surgical removal of the breast, axillary nodes, and chest muscles. Rarely performed anymore.

Hippocrates Institute: A Boston-based health education center emphasizing raw foods and juices.

histopathology: Abnormal appearance of cells. Different forms of breast cancer (like ductal and lobular) represent different histopathologies.

Hoxsey treatment: An herbal cancer treatment practiced in Mexico.

in situ *tumor:* A small, completely localized, confined tumor.

indole-3-carbinol: An anti-estrogenic substance found in cruciferous vegetables.

infiltrating: Invading the tissue immediately surrounding the tumor.

infiltrating ductal carcinoma: The most common form of breast cancer. See *infiltrating* and *ductal*.

isothiocyanates: A group of chemicals thought to have anticancer activity. Found in cruciferous vegetables.

laetrile: A variation on an isolate found in apricot pits. A once-popular alternative cancer treatment that appears ineffective. See *metabolic therapy.*

leucovorin: An activated form of the B vitamin folic acid.

lobular carcinoma: A type of breast cancer arising from lobules in the breast.

local recurrence: Return of cancer to the remaining breast or chest wall.

lignan: A fiber reported to have anti-estrogenic activity. Flaxseed is the best source.

Livingston-Wheeler Clinic: A San Diego-based alternative clinic that views cancer as an infection to be treated through the immune system.

lumpectomy: Surgical removal of a breast tumor and small amount of surrounding healthy tissue.

lycopene: An antioxidant found in tomatoes.

lymph nodes: Glands found in the armpit (axilla) and other parts of the body that function as part of the immune system. Breast cancer may spread to axillary nodes.

macrobiotic diet: A philosophically determined eating plan emphasizing brown rice, vegetables, and soy products and excluding red meat, poultry, eggs, and dairy products.

malignant: Cancerous.

mastectomy: Removal of the breast.

menarche: The time of the first menstrual cycle.

menopausal status: Whether the patient is pre- or postmenopausal.

meta-analysis: The pooling of data from previous research reports to create one large study. Meta-analyses may uncover important relationships not found in smaller studies.

metabolic therapy: An alternative cancer treatment that includes laetrile, enzymes, supplements, and dietary changes.

melatonin: A hormone secreted in the brain; it regulates sleep and may have anticancer activity.

metastatic: Having spread to another organ of the body.

methotrexate: A chemotherapy drug.

micrometastasis: Microscopic, undetectable pockets of cancer cells that have spread outside the breast.

modified radical mastectomy: Removal of the breast and axillary lymph nodes.

naturopathy: A medical system based on helping the body to heal itself using natural substances and noninvasive techniques. Naturopathic doctors are licensed in seven states and several Canadian provinces.

negative test result: Result is normal.

nodal sampling: Removing some but not all axillary lymph nodes.

node negative: No evidence of cancer in lymph nodes.

node positive: Cancer has been found in lymph nodes.

NSABP: National Surgical Adjuvant Breast and Bowel Project — a major American breast cancer research group.

oncologist: A medical doctor who is a cancer specialist.

ovarian ablation: Chemical or radiation-induced destruction or surgical removal of ovaries.

overall survival: Includes breast cancer survivors who have not suffered a recurrence plus those who have but remain alive.

pathologist: A medical doctor who specializes in the examination of biopsied tissue.

phytoestrogens: Substances found in plants that bear a structural resemblance to estrogen. Some may have anti-estrogenic activity.

ploidy status: Whether cancer cells have the appropriate number of chromosomes (diploid) or an abnormal number (aneuploid).

polyphenols: A group of antioxidants found in several edible plants. Some are thought to have anticancer activity.

positive test result: Result is abnormal.

postmenopausal: No longer having a menstrual cycle.

premenopausal: Still having a menstrual cycle. Having not yet gone through the menopause.

primary prevention: Preventing breast cancer in a woman who has never had the disease.

progestin: A synthetic drug with actions related to the female sex hormone progesterone.

prognosis: Expected outcome.

prospective study: A research design where subjects are investigated with blood tests, questions, etc., and then followed for years until some people develop the disease in question. Researchers then sift through the original information to see what separates those who eventually got sick from those who remained healthy.

quartile: 25 percent.

quintile: 20 percent.

recurrence: A return of cancer.

retrospective study: A research design where some subjects already have a disease and others don't. Both groups are asked about past behavior, nutrition, lifestyles, etc., in order to find which items distinguish the two groups.

S-phase fraction: The percentage of cancer cells synthesizing more cancer cells at a given moment.

screening mammogram: Mammogram done on a woman with no palpable lump and no obvious sign of breast cancer; done at regular intervals.

secondary prevention: Preventing a breast cancer recurrence.

shark cartilage: An alternative cancer treatment purported to interfere with a tumor's blood supply.

simple mastectomy: Removal of the breast.

stage: Indicates the size of the cancer and how far it has spread.

stage I: Small (2 cm or less) cancerous breast tumor with no cancer in lymph nodes.

stage II: Small tumor with limited cancer found in lymph nodes or a tumor over 2 cm in size with no cancer in lymph nodes.

sulforaphane: An anticancer substance found in broccoli.

systemic: Pertaining to the whole body.

tamoxifen: An estrogen-blocking drug (not chemotherapy).

thromboembolic: Pertaining to obstruction of blood vessels from excessive blood clotting.

type I error: When researchers or doctors mistakenly accept a useless therapy due to an association that resulted from chance.

type II error: When researchers or doctors mistakenly discard a useful therapy because of a lack of sufficient statistical proof.

ultrasound: See *diagnostic ultrasound.*

WBC: White blood cell — part of the body's immune system.

xenoestrogen: Non-natural substances that have estrogenic activity.

Index

300

INDEX

Anemia, 21, 27
Aneuploidy, 24–25
Angell, Marcia, 48
Angiogenesis, 131–132
Antioxidants, 141, 193, 196, 239. *See also individual antioxidants*
 dose, 223
 food sources, 288–290
 macrobiotic diet, 137
 and prevention, 211–223
Anxiety, with chemotherapy, 71
Appetite, loss of, with fluorouracil, 70
Aspiration cytology, 15–16
 in diagnosis flow chart, 12
 false negative result, 16
Aspirin, drug interactions, 70
Asthma, and tamoxifen, 115
Attitude, improved by intervention, 148
Avocados, 186
Axillary dissection, 17–20, 41, 108. *See also* Nodal sampling
 Cathy's decision, 58–59

Barberry, 138
Bastyr College, 140
Baum, Michael, 64
Beans, 168, 192
Beef, 180, 198
Beer, nonalcoholic, 236
Beta-carotene, 162, 167, 212
 deficiency, 219
 dose, 220
 food sources, 289
 Gerson therapy, 135
 and prevention, 218–220
Biomedical Center, Mexico, 139
Biopsy, 15–20. *See also individual procedures*
 aspiration cytology, 15–16
 in Cathy's story, 8
 excision, 8n, 17
 lumpectomy, 16–17
 unnecessary, 15
Birth control pills, 244–248
Birth defects
 and chemotherapy, 68–70
 and electric blankets, 249
Bisphenol-A, 250

Bladder, bleeding inflammation, with chemotherapy, 68, 71
Bladder cancer, with cyclophosphamide, 68
Bleeding, gastrointestinal, with fluorouracil, 70
Blood clotting disorders, with tamoxifen, 112
Blood tests, 20–21
 CBC (complete blood count), 21
 chem screen (SMAC), 21
 genetic screen, 26
Bonadonna, Gianni, 78, 89
Bone enzyme, 27
Bone scan, 26–27
Bowman-Birk protease inhibitor, 196, 227
Boyd, N. F., 174
BRCA1, 26, 121
Bread, 192, 261
Breast Cancer Prevention Trial, 118–122
Breast feeding. *See* Lactation
Breast implants, 47–48
Breast milk, and chemotherapy, 68. *See also* Lactation
Breast reconstruction, 47–49
Broccoli, 167, 194
Bross, Irwin, 49
Brussels sprouts, 194
Burish, Thomas, 68
Butter, 182, 225, 261

Cabbage, 194
Caffeine, 150, 237–238. *See also* Coffee; Tea
Calcium, 183
 macrobiotic diet, 136
Calculi, renal, 183, 261
 and vitamin C, 146
Caloric intake
 and breast cancer, 175–176
 reducing, 180
Cameron, Ewan, 142–143
Camoriano, Dr. John, 72
Cancer. *See individual types of cancer;* Carcinoma; Tumor
The Cancer Industry (Moss), 130n

About the Authors

Steve Austin, N.D., practices at the center for Natural Medicine in Portland, Oregon. Previously he was Professor of Nutrition at National College of Naturopathic Medicine and Assistant Professor at Western States Chiropractic College. He is an internationally respected speaker in the field of clinical nutrition.

Dr. Austin holds bachelor's degrees in psychology from Antioch College and human biology from Kansas Newman College. He graduated from National College of Naturopathic Medicine in 1982. He is a licensed naturopathic physician. Naturopathic physicians employ conventional diagnostic procedures but treat patients with nutrition, supplements, herbs, manipulation, and other natural therapies.

Dr. Austin is a contributor to *A Textbook of Natural Medicine* and on the editorial board of *The Journal of Naturopathic Medicine.* His research on alternative cancer clinics in Mexico appears in the May 1994 issue of *The Journal of Naturopathic Medicine.* Many naturopathic, medical, and chiropractic physicians in the United States and Canada follow Dr. Austin's newsletter *Clinical Nutrition Update.*

Cathy Hitchcock, M.S.W., is a licensed clinical social worker in private practice. She received her bachelor's degree in education from the University of Washington and her M.S.W. from Portland State University in 1984.

Although her general counseling practice includes both men and women, Ms. Hitchcock's professional focus has historically been on women's issues such as molestation, body image, eating disorders, and female sexuality. She leads an ongoing women's therapy group and sees both individuals and couples in her practice.

Ms. Hitchcock also counsels individuals suffering from chronic or life-threatening diseases. She uses her experience as a breast cancer patient to help some clients make the transition to empowered survivors, while others she helps with death and dying issues.